Strong Bones Forever

*The Complete Drug-Free System for
Preventing and Reversing
Osteoporosis Using Diet, Exercise,
Lifestyle, and Supplementation*

Contents

1

Introduction

In May 2018 researchers in Barcelona reported the results of a case study on one of the world's oldest living humans. It was determined that at the ripe old age of 113 this man had a perfect skeleton. His bones were of normal density and curvature and, additionally, showed no abnormalities that could be expected for someone of his advanced years. Most importantly, he had never broken a bone. Researchers then performed genetic testing in an attempt to discover the "magic gene" that was responsible for his longevity and strong bones. What they found was nothing short of astounding!

His genes were ... absolutely average. They could find no such magic gene.

Further investigation revealed that one factor could not be considered average and may have contributed greatly to his longevity and strong skeleton: the man's lifestyle. He had led a very healthy and active life, which included eating a classic Mediterranean diet and being extraordinarily active even by standards for someone 20 years younger.

There are two important takeaways here:

· Poor lifestyle is the cause of most cases of osteoporosis, rather than poor genetics.

· The health of the bones is a fairly accurate indication of the health of the rest of the body.

This appears to be more than just mere correlation: bones play a central role in regulating key nutrients, hormones, and minerals that have an impact on the health of the brain and cardiovascular system.

The bottom line? Success leaves clues. In the chapters that follow, you will learn precisely what you need to do to enjoy STRONG BONES FOR LIFE. So, buckle up because it is going to be quite a ride. You will have to read with an open mind as I report on study after study that flies in the face of conventional medicine.

You have nothing to lose by reading with an open mind—but you have much to lose if you refuse to take this journey. What could you lose? It starts with your bones and ends with your independence, your very freedom to explore and to travel and to enjoy life to its fullest. I truly want you to live your fullest life without fear that your bones will break. I want you to be the envy of your friends as you age, rather than ending up hunched over and fragile. I never want you to be dependent on the care of loved ones, friends, or strangers in white coats. That is the legacy that I hope to leave through the information in this book.

2

Quick Start Guide

Begin Today! Start Building Bone Right Now!

I have designed this book to answer every conceivable question that you may have regarding bone health, osteopenia, and osteoporosis. I have intentionally kept the book as focused and concentrated as possible in order to facilitate action. With that said, I realize that even a quick read can be difficult to fit into the hustle and bustle of everyday life. So I have included this quick-start guide to get you underway today, at this very moment, to provide your body with the nutrients and stimulus to begin growing new, healthy, pliable bone.

Below, you will find my general recommendations, which will be refined and become more advanced as the book goes on. But, for now, let us get started with the six simple steps listed below.

STEP 1: Look at Your Current Calcium Formula

One fundamental philosophy of this program is to choose a **BONE MINERAL FORMULA** that contains calcium, along with magnesium, boron, silica, and other trace minerals. I have provided a list of supplements from which to choose; some are available in local health-food stores, while others can be purchased on the internet. As you will learn in the coming chapters, calcium alone is not enough to build healthy bones. To strengthen the skeleton, you need numerous building blocks, so start thinking in terms of bone minerals rather than calcium. For an updated list of supplements I

recommend, visit
OsteoCoach.com/StrongBonesForever.

STEP 2: Take At Least 2,000 IU Of Vitamin D3 (Cholecalciferol)

Ingesting 2,000 International Units (IU) of vitamin D_3 (cholecalciferol) is a very safe dosage. If you are taking prescription vitamin D, skip this step until you read Chapter 6. You may then want to revisit this issue with your doctor once you are armed with that new information. Doses up to 4,000 IU are considered safe for most people. *Never choose vitamin D_2 (ergocalciferol) as this is an inferior formula.* Most people find the dose that raises their blood levels to the optimal range is between 2,000 and 5,000 IU per day.

STEP 3: Eat As Many Green Leafy Vegetables As You Can Fit Into Your Diet.

These vegetables are especially beneficial for bones because they provide the alkaline compounds that feed bone-building cells and prevent bone erosion. Although we will get into the topic of building a bone-friendly diet in a future chapter, for now, simply ramp up the vegetables. I recommend a minimum of five servings per day, ideally 8 to10 servings.

STEP 4: Purchase a Weighted Vest and Go for a Walk While Wearing It

You control the amount of weight in these vests, available at such retailers as Walmart The added weight adds load to bones, which can help stabilize bone loss and may even help you gain a little more bone mass over time. While you are shopping, you may also want to buy walking poles for stability.

STEP 5: Supplement With Vitamin K

As you will learn, Vitamin D assists in carrying various minerals into the bloodstream, while vitamin K tells the body where to deposit those minerals. If your goal is to draw calcium into the blood and keep it out of the arteries, then you need to make sure to take the daily recommended dietary allowance (RDA) of vitamin K. The only contraindication (or inadvisability) for vitamin K pertains to people who take Coumadin® or warfarin, its generic equivalent. Since Coumadin/warfarin thins the blood and vitamin K helps to clot the blood, the two work against each other in the body. Therefore, if you take Coumadin/warfarin, skip this step.

STEP 6: Lift Weights

The research clearly establishes that when you expose the body to carrying heavy loads, bones get stronger. This is evident in bodybuilders and gymnasts, who tend to have extraordinarily strong bones. You do not need to be a bodybuilder or gymnast, however, to improve your bone strength by lifting heavier weights two to three times per week. For now, just get into the habit of lifting weights on a regular basis and I will cover specific ways to optimize your exercise for strengthening bones later in the book. Depending on your situation, you may not yet be ready for this step. That is okay! Later in the book we will provide more particulars on building a healthy workout plan. If you are located near Baltimore, Maryland, there is a center devoted to helping people achieve the needed stimulus to build bones in just 7 to 10 minutes, performed once a week. Find out more details at OsteoCoach.com .If you are not in the Baltimore area, you may be able to find a center offering the BioDensity workout by visiting BioDensity.com.

3

How Your Bones Work

Here are the facts from the National Osteoporosis Foundation website:

·Worldwide, there is an osteoporotic fracture every 3 seconds

·10 million Americans have osteoporosis—80% are women

- 34 million Americans have low Bone Mass
- 18 million Americans have osteopenia ("pre-osteoporosis")
- One in three women over 50 will suffer an osteoporosis-related fracture in their life
- One in five men over 50 will suffer an osteoporosis-related fracture in their

life

- Osteoporosis is the cause of 1.5 million fractures annually
- In 1995, osteoporosis-related fractures cost Americans $38 million PER DAY

Although these numbers seem daunting, I like to point out that there is a great deal of hype about osteoporosis. Pharmaceutical companies that make medicines to treat osteoporosis—discussed in detail later—fuel some of this hype. What is important to note is that the skeleton is as vital an organ as the heart or liver. It needs to be nourished, cared for, and used but not abused, or that structure will begin to crumble.

This book discusses what feeds and nourishes your skeleton so that you have the knowledge you need to have a strong and healthy frame for life!

Let us begin by exploring the prevalence and significance of osteoporosis …

During childhood and adolescence, bones are modeled into what ultimately develops into the adult skeleton. Then in adulthood a process of remodeling occurs where bones are constantly broken down and rebuilt. It is estimated that, on average, 10 percent of bone is removed and rebuilt every year, resulting in a brand-new skeleton approximately every decade.

What The Heck Is Going On Here?

Not long ago, scientists discovered the bones of what came to be known as our oldest "human-ish" relative, lovingly referred to as Lucy. After carbon dating, it was determined that Lucy's skeleton is over 3.2 million years old. That is right: 3.2 million years after Lucy's death we were still able to dig up and recognize her bones.

Does anyone else see something wrong with this?

Every other tissue in Lucy's entire body disintegrated … except her bones. Why are we having trouble preventing our bones from disintegrating within our own bodies while Lucy's skeleton can tell us a story 3.2 million years later?

This is a fair question, right?

In a nutshell, the human body has never before, in its 3.2-plus-million years of existence, been subjected to the chemicals, calories, and "Franken-foods" that it is exposed to in modern times. Never in the evolution of the human body has it enjoyed the luxury of having food delivered to its lap while exerting no more energy than to enjoy 5 or 6 hours of television per day. In an effort to conserve energy, the body removes tissues that are not being used—in this case, bones.

The Theory Behind Our Crumbling Structure

Bone structure can be equated to a large skyscraper constantly undergoing structural maintenance. One team of workers tears down old, failing walls, while another team erects new, stronger walls. Our bones have cells, called osteoclasts, that break down old, brittle bone; they also have osteoblasts that build new, strong, pliable bone where the old, brittle bone was removed.

In our youth, these teams of cells work hard, although osteoblasts (bone builders) work harder than osteoclasts (bone removers), to make our bones strong. This equates to building a skyscraper from the ground up, and when the skyscraper is completed, retaining just enough workers to maintain the structure.

Now, imagine that it requires more energy and building blocks to erect structures than it does to break them down, and you have a working model of what happens to bones as you age. For some reason, bone builders begin to work less efficiently than bone removers, resulting in more bone breakdown than bone building, with the end result being the structure (bone) grows weaker and begins to crumble.

In forthcoming sections, we will discuss some of the reasons bone builders slow production, as well as why we have fewer bone builders as we age.

It is important to note that bone removers do not just chomp up the old, brittle bone; clock out; and head home for the day. As they move through the bone, they leave a trail of compounds called growth factors that attract and stimulate the bone builders to fill in gaps with new bone. The vitally important takeaway here is that anything poisoning these bone removers will also poison the bone builders and thus prevent the formation of healthy, strong, pliable bone.

Bone structure is comprised of two types of bone material: cortical bone and trabecular bone and cortical bone. The cortical bone surrounds the trabecular bone as a dense outer shell, and the honeycomb-like trabecular bone gives bone its amazing strength.

Osteoporosis most commonly occurs in the trabecular bone, which is found in higher quantities in bones most likely to fracture, such as the hips, spine, and forearms. (Osteoporotic fractures can occur in any bone, but those listed above are the most incapacitating.) Osteoporotic bone viewed under a microscope shows a disappearance of the honeycomb shape that ultimately becomes excessively porous.

Silent fractures (fractures that show on X-ray despite the patient having no pain or symptoms) in the spine can lead to the characteristic loss of height and humpback appearance associated with osteoporosis. The "osteoporotic hump," as it is known in the medical community, also forces the posture into a forward-leaning position that increases the risk of falls with the resulting catastrophic fractures of the hip and/or thighbone (femur).

Reaching Your Peak Bone Mass

This section is of utmost importance to those either being under age 30 or having loved ones under 30. Bone mineral density increases from infancy through adolescence and peaks around age 30. After that time, bone density levels out and begins a slow, steady decline of between 1 to 2 percent per year until menopause, when it increases to 3 to 5 percent bone loss per year, according to a 2010 report of the International Osteoporosis Foundation. Therefore, it is important to be active and live a healthy lifestyle in younger years, since the higher the bone density when reaching your peak the more bone can be lost before you become osteoporotic. To illustrate, imagine taking a helicopter to the peak of a mountain and then being instructed to walk back down. The higher the peak of the mountain, the longer it will take to reach the bottom. There are many factors that affect how high your peak is.

Factors That Affect Peak Bone as We Develop:

- Mineral content of the diet (calcium, magnesium, etc.)
- Vitamin D levels throughout adolescence
- Adequate physical activity
- Refraining from excessive physical activity
- Smoking history
- Alcohol intake
- Vegetable intake

- Amount of stress in your life
- Intake of soda and other acidifying foods
- Adequate protein intake
- Use of medications that inhibit bone
- Early menopause (whether surgical or natural)
- History of rheumatoid arthritis
- Use of proton pump inhibitors (PPIs)

The research is clear that adequate mineral intake throughout adolescence is a critical factor in determining how strong and dense bones are leading up to the 30s. Sadly, many doctors still believe that after peak mass is reached bones cannot grow stronger without pharmaceutical intervention, such as Fosamax® or Actonel®. Although bones do not grow longer, they can grow stronger with the right lifestyle shifts—no matter your age. In fact, there are numerous cases in which bones have grown literally stronger when adequate nutrition is maintained and stimulation is applied through the right type of exercise. In addition to personal observation, numerous studies have demonstrated the amazing ability of bones to grow stronger even in later years when such osteogenic stimulation is applied. In this book, you will learn principles that will help strengthen your bones no matter how weak they are and how many years you have logged.

Will you be able to achieve the same bone density you had when you were 20? Probably not. It appears that bones decrease in density with age, but this does not necessarily translate into a weakened bone structure. In other words, a high bone density does not guarantee that you will not suffer an osteoporotic fracture and a low bone density does not guarantee that you will. The aim is not to only fix some arbitrary number in your medical records, such as your DXA score (bone density test), but rather to enjoy strong bones and a lifetime free from an osteoporotic fracture. This is achievable even if your bone density never reaches the density of your 20s or 30s.

Menopause and Bone Loss

Now, let us tackle the midyears when menopause comes into play. There is no questioning the connection between menopause and increased bone loss, but it is important to note that all postmenopausal years are not created equal. Refer back to the section regarding how bones are constantly being broken down and rebuilt. As mentioned earlier, when bone is worn down or damaged through everyday activity, the bone-removing cells move in and clear out the old, brittle bone. As they clean up the damaged bone, they signal the bone-building cells to refill the pits with new and healthy bone.

After menopause, the pits left by the bone-removing cells are deeper and the work done by the bone-building cells is not quite as efficient, so the architecture of the bone is of lower quality. Estrogen plays an important role in regulating the birth of new bone-removing cells by blocking a compound that turns osteoclast precursor cells into active bone-removing cells, which makes it easier to produce bone-removing cells after the onset of menopause. With time, this incomplete or "shoddy" work caused by sluggish bone-building cells, along with the existence of more bone-removing cells, can lead to porous bone that develops into osteoporosis.

The first three to six years after menopause are critical to the strength of your postmenopausal bones after menopause as bone loss occurs at a much higher rate and then levels off to premenopausal levels. Unfortunately, during this period of aggressive bone loss, many women may lose up to 20 percent of their bone mass. Controlling certain factors that accelerate this loss of bone is critical; although those influences are important during your entire life, extra care should be taken during this six or seven years postmenopausal period. These factors include smoking habits, alcohol use, exercise and activity level, certain pharmaceuticals, stress, diet, and supplementation. These factors will be covered in more depth later in the book.

What Fixes Your Bones, Fixes Your Body

Remember the old song that went through each bone in the human body and how it is connected to other bones? Well, it turns out that the connection goes far beyond a bone-to-bone relationship.

The same actions that keep bones healthy also keep the other organs and muscles working properly. For example, even though minerals comprise less than one half of one percent of brain volume, without those minerals the brain would not function at all. When the brain is deficient in such minerals as calcium, magnesium, and zinc, it becomes sluggish, resulting in poor memory and function. As you put the recommendations to follow into action, you will find that you are feeling and thinking better well before your bones start showing discernable improvements. Consider it icing on the cake!

Thyroid: A New Perspective

For anyone diagnosed with a thyroid condition, you are probably most interested in this section. It is, however, an important section for everyone to read because recent research has changed the way the thyroid's role in the health of bone is viewed. Unfortunately, your doctor may not be familiar with this new research, and you will need to advocate for yourself.

It is no secret that bones are at risk when the thyroid hormones are higher than normal. If you take a prescription thyroid hormone—such as Synthroid®, Levoxyl®, or Armour® Thyroid—then you are already aware of this fact because your doctor is very cautious about dosage. You likely get regular blood tests to evaluate your level of the thyroid stimulating hormone (TSH), which is true to its name. When the body senses that the thyroid hormone called thyroxine (T4) is low, the body produces TSH to get the thyroid to release more of that thyroid hormone. If the thyroid is dysfunctional, then the gland produces either too little thyroxine (which results in hypothyroidism) or produces too much thyroid hormone (which results in hyperthyroidism). If you are diagnosed with an under-active thyroid, then you have likely been prescribed one of the previously mentioned hormone medications with the goal to get the TSH down as much as possible, while additionally treating any symptoms you may have, such as fatigue, thinning hair, intolerance to cold, "foggy mind," and dry skin.

Medicine views TSH as nothing more than a hormone that is responsible for communicating how much thyroid hormone (thyroxine) is present in the body. The current medical belief is that TSH has no other effect on the body. However, nature is not that inefficient; it turns out that TSH is utilized as a means of communicating with the bone-removing and bone-building cells of the body.

Researchers recently discovered that when TSH is too low (as is the case in hyperthyroidism or when too much thyroid medication is taken), the bone-building cells work slower and the bone-removing cells work overtime.

Unfortunately, when TSH is too high the same outcome occurs. As with anything related to health, the body craves balance (*J Bone Miner Res.* 2007 June 22(6):849–59).

So what does this mean for you?

There are two main messages here: First, if you are currently being treated for hypothyroidism, request that your doctor keep the TSH within a healthy range but not excessively low. Second, if you are currently not being treated for hypothyroidism, then it is worthwhile for you to keep your thyroid healthy in order to protect your bones. By follo

So what does this mean for you?

There are two main messages here: First, if you are currently being treated for hypothyroidism, request that your doctor keep the TSH within a healthy range but not excessively low. Second, if you are currently not being treated for hypothyroidism, then it is worthwhile for you to keep your thyroid healthy in order to protect your bones. By following the dietary and exercise advice in this book, you should be well protected.

Chapter Summary:

It is estimated that the human body makes approximately 1.75 million bone cells every second. That equates to 150 billion new bone-building cells every single day. The quality and function of those cells will be determined by the quality and quantity of materials that the body has available. The goal of a healthy bone-building program is to provide superior building blocks in sufficient quantity to build fully functioning, high-quality cells and then to activate them with proper lifestyle and nutrition. Once this happens, your body will have the tools to repair your bone matrix and to enjoy healthy, strong bones for life. Now that you have a fundamental understanding of how bones work, let us get into more functional details, such as how to test your bones and how to reverse osteoporosis.

4

How Your Bones Shrink and Grow

Chapter 1 presented you with basic knowledge of how bones are built in the human body. In this chapter, you will hone in on proper daily upkeep of bones after density has peaked, around age 30. By the end of this chapter, you should understand why you have lost bone over the years and will be able to lay the groundwork for stabilizing and eventually restoring lost bone.

To review, there are two core bone cells that are important to the upkeep of our skeleton: osteoblasts (bone builders) and osteoclasts (bone removers). We have already discussed how the bone-removing cells eat the damaged and old bone and leave a "breadcrumb trail" of growth factors that cause bone builders to fill in any pits left in the bone. As the bone builders fill in new bone, some get trapped in the matrix and turn into cells called osteocytes. Osteocytes are very important to the process of building new bone, and we will cover them in this chapter.

Bone is composed of two main components: bone cells and the "extracellular matrix" discussed below. As we examined earlier, bone cells are made up of osteoclasts and osteoblasts (osteocytes are a form of bone-building cell). The extracellular matrix is made up of organic and inorganic materials. The organic material is made up of type I collagen, proteins, and proteoglycans that form the scaffolding on which the minerals are laid. The inorganic materials are mainly calcium and phosphorous, and to lesser degrees magnesium, potassium, and trace minerals. This will become important as we get into the types of foods and supplements needed to protect and to produce new bone.

After bone density peaks, bone remodeling (the process of eating old bone and laying new bone, as discussed in Chapter 1) goes through four phases:

- Phase 1: Activation (work order issued)
- Phase 2: Resorption (demolition of old structure)
- Phase 3: Formation (building new structure)
- Phase 4: Resting (work complete; awaiting new work order)

When in the course of everyday living small microfractures occur in bone, a work order—called RANKL (receptor activator of nuclear factor kappa-B ligand)—is sent out to call in the bone-removing cells. RANKL causes baby bone-removing cells to turn into adult bone-removing cells that then go out and eat up the damaged area. Certain factors can trigger RANKL to be secreted by stromal cells in the marrow, such as parathyroid hormone (PTH), inflammatory compounds, and certain prostaglandins. Interestingly, estrogen causes stromal cells to produce a compound that blocks RANKL from doing its job, which is why estrogen is so beneficial to bones. By blocking RANKL, baby bone-removing cells do not grow into adult cells and the bone-breaking process slows down. Estrogen thus acts as a failsafe to prevent excess activation of bone-removing cells resulting in a balance of bone removal and bone repair. Once activated, the bone-removing cells bind to the bone wall and secrete acid to remove minerals and enzymes to dissolve collagen and protein to remove the old bone in a process called resorption. The liberated minerals and protein are sent into the bloodstream to be recycled or excreted. <u>The resorption process takes three to four weeks to complete.</u>

Once the damaged bone is removed, bone-removing cells disappear through a natural and healthy process of programmed cell suicide and stem cells are converted into osteoblasts, the bone builders that lay down new bone in the third phase called formation. <u>Although bone resorption takes three to four weeks,</u> <u>it is important to note that bone formation takes more time and resources,</u> <u>up to three to four months to complete.</u>

As bone-building cells lay down new bone, some bone builders voluntarily trap themselves in the new bone and form a network of interconnected cells called osteocytes or "mechanoreceptors," which monitor bone for stress and damage. This is a vital process in the production of new bone. When these osteocytes sense damage or stress to bone, they send out activation signals that trigger resorption and then formation. In essence, osteocytes act as the foreman cells of the bone and are responsible for sending orders to osteoclasts and osteoblasts.

Once bone is remodeled, it enters the resting phase in which bone cells go dormant while awaiting a new work order.

Let me bottom line this for you so you know why I felt it important to explain this somewhat complex process:

1. The idea that all we humans need to do is throw calcium at bones and they will grow stronger is misguided —not to mention just plain wrong. Bone building is a highly regulated process that requires much more than calcium to improve the skeleton. For example, no work order, no bone building regardless of how much calcium you take.
2. Estrogen is a useful tool in keeping bone-removing cells in line. In the right amount, forms, and situation, it can be a game-changer by controlling RANKL and thus the number of adult bone-removing cells.
3. Bones are made up of far more than minerals; collagen, protein, and proteoglycans are also important components.
4. There are four phases of the remodeling process, each dependent on the other in a sequential fashion. Drugs focus exclusively on the suppression of the resorption phase, ignoring that without resorption, the process of formation becomes hobbled. Without activation,

resorption *and* formation become sluggish and inefficient.

5. Osteocytes could be the rate-limiting factor in building healthy bone because they are responsible for sending the work orders to activate bone remodeling.

6. The bottom of the bottom line? Osteoporosis is no more a calcium deficiency than it is a Fosamax deficiency. Although both can slow down the demineralization of bone, neither will strengthen your bone. We must take a strategic approach to building bone that influences all four phases of the bone-formation process.

To successfully build new bone, you need a comprehensive system for optimizing the activation, resorption, and formation of new bone. That is what we are here to do!

In the next chapter, we will cover the DXA scan, which is considered the gold standard method for assessing and monitoring the status of bones.

5

Understanding Your Bone Scans

The DXA Scan – What is it?

Getting bone density tested is a simple and painless process, which usually involves the use of some sort of X-ray testing equipment. There are two main types of tests: central and peripheral. Central testing evaluates the bone density of the spine, hips, and total body; peripheral testing evaluates the density of the wrists, kneecaps, shinbones, and heels. Recently, tests have been approved to evaluate bone density through a test of finger bones; however, there are questions as to how useful this is for evaluating risk for developing osteoporosis. The gold standard scan is called dual X-Ray absorptiometry, or DXA (pronounced "Dexa"), which evaluates the spine, hips, and total body.

When you receive your bone density test results, you will see two different scores: one compared with "young-normal" and the other with "age-matched norms." The young-normal, also called the T-score, compares your results with those of a healthy 30-year-old adult. The age-matched norm, also known as the Z-score, compares your results with what is expected for someone of your age and body frame. However, since older folks have a tendency toward lower bone density, the Z-score can be somewhat misleading. The T-score gives the best representation of fracture risk, which increases as bone density decreases further from the young-normal range. Upcoming is a table that further explains the significance of the T-score. We will then discuss the shortcomings of the DXA scan.

As it pertains to osteoporosis, the statistical term "standard deviation" is used to describe how far a person's bone density is from the majority of the "healthy population." For each 1.0 standard deviation below the young adult mean, your bone density has decreases decreased 10 to 12 percent below the norm. It is not important that you understand the statistical significance of standard deviation, only what it means in your risk of fracture. So if you are 3.0 standard deviations below the young adult mean (which would be indicated as -3.0 on the DXA report), your density is approximately 30 to 36 percent lower than normal. It has been estimated that for every 10 percent decrease in bone density your fracture risk doubles. This all seems cut and dried—however, in actuality, it is far from a foregone conclusion.

T-Score Range

Normal Density

No increased risk of fracture
Within 1 SD (0 to -1 standard deviation)
(Standard deviation)

Osteopenia

No increased risk of fracture
-1 to -2.5 SD
(Standard deviation)

Osteopenia

Some bone loss, mild risk
-2.5 Sd or more
(Standard deviation)

Osteoporosis

Significantly increased risk of fracture
-2.5 Sd & one or more fracture
(standard deviation)
Severe established Osteoporosis

Two Main Forms of Osteoporosis

It is important to note that there are two types of osteoporosis: primary and secondary. Primary osteoporosis is the bone loss that is commonly associated with aging and menopause, and is found in otherwise healthy people. Most doctors consider primary osteoporosis to be a natural progression in bone loss from age (although I would disagree).

Secondary osteoporosis refers to bone loss that is attributed to something other than age-associated bone loss. Secondary bone loss, which can happen in younger men and women, usually has a discernible cause, such as steroid use, hyperthyroid, rheumatoid arthritis, celiac disease, PPIs (reflux medications), etc. When assessing DXA scans in primary osteoporosis, the T-score is usually used to assess bone density. When evaluating bone loss in secondary osteoporosis, the Z-score may be a better place to look. This is especially the case in younger people (age 64 or younger). That being said, both scores are useful in evaluating and monitoring bone density.

What's Wrong with the DXA SCAN?

The DXA scan was developed to do one thing: determine the density (hardness) of bone. It does not determine the quality of bone being examined. Some researchers estimate that even if bone density in the spine decreases by 50 percent, it should still be architecturally able to withstand five times the strain it would normally be exposed to from everyday wear and tear. "How can that be?" you may ask. "Doesn't a low bone density mean you are at a high risk of fracture?" According to L. Joseph Melton III, MD of the Mayo Clinic, "Osteoporosis alone may not be sufficient to produce a fracture since many individuals remain fracture-free even within the subgroups with the lowest bone density. Most women aged sixty-five and over and men seventy-five and over have lost enough bone to place them at a significant risk of osteoporotic fracture, yet many never fracture any bones at all. By age eighty virtually all women in the United States are osteoporotic with regard to hip bone density, yet only a small percentage of them suffer hip fractures each year" (Harvard University Continuing Education Course on Osteoporosis, 1987).

Allow me to let you in on the way that the research world works: Medical scientists are always looking for grants from various companies so that they can do what they love to do most, which is study stuff. These researchers are often funded by the same companies that make the drug that they are studying. Therefore, there's impetus to find and publish positive findings and to simultaneously sweep negative findings "under the rug". To satisfy the company that provides the grant, they often choose to study the things that are most likely to paint the product being studied in a positive light. This way, when the study is complete, the same company will want to give them more money to study more stuff.

In osteoporosis research, the easiest thing to study is bone density. The studies can be done rather quickly and, because the current model of osteoporosis exists under the premise that density determines fracture risk, they can extrapolate an improvement in density to mean benefits to fracture risk. As you probably can tell by now, I am not a fan of density as the sole marker of fracture risk. I want to know how a variable impacts "Break-Rates." In other words, does a particular product (drug/supplement/diet/tool/type of exercise) decrease the risk of breaking a bone? An increase in density means nothing to me if the quality of bone suffers. The current research model is a despicable practice. Yes, it does promote research—but who cares if the research being produced is rancid with bias?

A large-scale study in 1998 investigated 9,700 women, 443 of whom suffered hip fractures over a 9-year period. Of these 443 women, just 57 percent had low bone density; 27 percent had medium bone density, and 16 percent had high bone density. Clearly, bone density is not the only factor in determining fracture risk. If it were the only important variable, then how is it that a full 43 percent of the women who suffered a hip fracture—a characteristic sign of osteoporosis—had medium to high bone density? Susan E. Brown, PhD, in her book *Better Bones Better Body,* formulates a new equation for determining osteoporosis risk.

The New Formula:

Thin Osteoporotic Bone (Low Density) + Poor Bone Self-Repair = Bone Fracture Risk

What this means is that the disease of osteoporosis cannot be diagnosed simply by looking at bone density. The quality of bone present and its ability to repair and rebuild when damaged also has to be taken into account. You are going to learn how conventional approaches to treating osteoporosis violate this formula by affecting only one part (density) and ignoring the more important factor of bone quality.

In fact, as mentioned previously, when medications poison the bone-removing cells, then bone repair and the rejuvenation process are also poisoned. This is why a grossly negative impact on bone fracture risk is expected with long-term treatment using conventional drugs, such as Fosamax, Boniva®, and Actonel. More on this later ...

Certainly bone density is an important factor in the risk for osteoporotic fracture, but the take-home message is that density is only one of many key factors. For example, bone quality is even more important than density. The pharmaceutical companies would love to have you believe that bone density is all that matters because, in truth, their drugs really impact only the density of bone. The net effect on "quality" of bone may be quite negative and even catastrophic, as demonstrated by an increase in risk of jaw necrosis and low-impact, spontaneous bone fractures in patients taking these medications for extended periods.

Poor Bone Self Repair – The Second Part of the Equation

Let us talk briefly about the second part of the equation: poor bone self-repair. It is almost entirely an artifact of lifestyle. However, age also plays a role, as was demonstrated in what I believe to be the most important study to date that you (and probably your doctor) have never heard about. It investigated 9,516 women ages 65 and older. Researchers set out to determine the most important factors associated with the risk of bone fracture. At the completion of the study, they were able to identify almost two dozen risk factors for bone fracture. Of those, 16 were found to significantly increase the risk of fracture independent of the women's bone density.

In other words, a woman could have normal bone density and still be at increased risk of osteoporotic fracture if she had a number of other risk factors. And if low bone density is included as a risk factor, then there are 17 main risk factors and six lesser factors.

It is extremely important that you understand that bone density was listed among the 17 risk factors and not *the sole risk factor* for osteoporosis. Unfortunately, your doctor probably never got wind of this study, despite the fact that it was published in one of the most reputable journals of the medical industry. Why? Simply because the drugs physicians prescribe can only influence one factor of the total 17.

Let us dive into some of these fascinating findings …

So, what are these risk factors? And what do you need to do about them? This is such an important finding that I decided to provide the checklist at the end of this chapter (*N Engl J Med* 332.12; 1995: 767–774). It will allow you to assess your bone quality as it pertains to the risk of fracture. By knowing the quality of your bones, you are able to decide how aggressive your personal osteoporosis plan needs to be in order to have a meaningful impact on lowering the risk of breaking a bone. It is so beneficial to have an easy tool that goes beyond bone density to help you ascertain your true risk. I hope that you are now beginning to see that—like many things in life—quality is more important than quantity. I want to help you build quality bone; the density will follow.

Risk Factors and Likelihood of Fracture

Women with two or fewer of the 16 risk factors that do not include low bone density had an incidence rate of hip fracture of 1.1 per 1,000 woman-years. That is astoundingly low. This accounted for approximately 47 percent of the study group.

Women with five or more risk factors not including low bone density had a hip fracture incidence of 19 per 1,000 woman-years. This accounted for 15 percent of the women studied. This is a fascinating finding because 15 percent of women were at significantly higher risk of osteoporotic fracture while still having a "normal" bone density.

Women with five or more risk factors in addition to a bone density in the lowest third for their age had a hip fracture incidence of 27 per 1,000 woman-years, a 27-fold increase in risk compared with the women with two or fewer risk factors. In addition, these women accounted for over one-third of hip fractures in the entire group.

More Proof That Density Is Only One Factor

When researchers evaluated fracture risk across age groups who share similar bone densities, they found that fracture risk was not equal between age groups. In other words, if the bone density was 0.70 gm/cm for a person between ages 60 and 64, the risk would be just 20 per 1,000 person-years. However, if someone between ages 75 and 79 had the same bone density, then the risk would be 60 per 1,000 person-years, or three times the risk. This just goes to show that bone density is just one factor and the quality or the bone is equally if not more important (*Journal of Clinical Investigation* 81, 1988). It also shows that, all things being equal, quality of bone suffers from age regardless of bone density. At the OsteoCoach Center for Strong Bones, we function on the proven premise that lifestyle can influence the rate of skeletal aging. So, as you improve your lifestyle, you also can protect and improve the quality *and* density of your bones.

What About the Screenings Available at the Local Grocery Store or Drug Store?

Quantitative ultrasound (QUS) measures bone density through the heel, using harmless radio waves instead of the X-rays used by a DXA machine. This test, designed for finding people at risk of osteoporosis, is limited by the fact that it, like DXA, measures only the density of the bones. QUS, unfortunately, is limited in that it cannot be used to monitor changes in bone density and a good score does not guarantee the person does not suffer from osteoporosis. In other words, if the score is low, you are likely to have bone thinning, but if your score is good it does not necessarily let you off the hook, as you may still have osteopenia or even osteoporosis in other bones. A DXA scan may still be needed for full evaluation, depending on your health history. Many experts in the osteoporosis field try to steer people away from "heel screening" due to the fact that it is relatively inaccurate compared with DXA scans.

There is newer technology in osteoporosis screening that uses updated technology to evaluate bones in arms, fingers, tibias (in the legs), and feet. This method, called Omnipath™ Axial Transmission Technology produced by BeamMed, appears to be much more precise and has even won U.S. Food and Drug Administration (FDA) approval for monitoring bone loss over time. The benefit of using this test is it is less expensive than administering a DXA scan and does not expose the patient to radiation. In addition, this technology can actually scan areas that are potential fracture risks, such as the forearm bone and the tibia. If you are considering undergoing screening, you may want to find a qualified professional in your area who uses the BeamMed Omnisense technology. Though it will not replace DXA, it could be a useful tool in monitoring your progress between DXA scans, as DXA scans are generally only performed every two years.

When Should You Consider Getting a DXA Scan?

There are two main answers to this question: one answer is for the general population, and the other is for people with "extenuating circumstances." Let us start with the extenuating circumstances.

Women who are premenopausal and do not have regular menstrual cycles or have been on long-term treatment with anticonvulsant medications, heartburn medications, or steroids should have a bone mass assessment done ASAP. In addition, women who currently have or have had eating disorders should also be evaluated. In these situations, it is very common for the process of bone loss to be significantly accelerated. If this is the case, it is better to know about it early so that an aggressive approach to improving the condition of bones—or at least the delay of progression to osteoporosis—can be undertaken.

For the general population, approaching menopause is an excellent time to get a bone mineral test. As mentioned earlier, there are many factors that determine personal peak bone mass. These variables result in a wide spectrum of bone densities, however, when you are lumped into statistical norms, which may not represent your personal risk. It is not uncommon for many women to have their bone density tested for the first time well after menopause, only to immediately be diagnosed with osteopenia or osteoporosis. Unfortunately, medicine has an alarmist response to such a result, which leads to aggressive treatment. One test alone cannot determine the "bone loss velocity," which is the rate of change in density. If a baseline test demonstrates your bone density showing osteopenia as you approach menopause, then 10 years later a result that shows little change from that previous test should not cause alarm because bone density is relatively stable. A lifestyle program can be formulated as opposed to resorting to prescribing toxic medications. In addition, anyone osteopenic or osteoporotic and approaching menopause can make more informed decisions about possible lifestyle changes through those initial six or seven years when bone loss is accelerated.

As reported earlier, the significance of bone density means different things at different ages. If you are 55 and osteoporotic, your risk of fracture is far less than someone who is 80 with an identical bone density. At age 55 you may not need to resort to osteoporosis drugs as your risk may still be relatively low and your capacity for movement and exercise is far greater than for that octogenarian. That does not mean being of an advanced age automatically necessitates your taking drugs, but the cards are a bit more stacked against you. More care will need to be taken in building an exercise plan and being diligent with supplements and other strategies.

From the perspective of fracture risk, DXA scans are only useful for people over age 65. The only reason to get a baseline DXA before age 65 is to determine a baseline, to assess the bone loss velocity, and/or to diagnose secondary osteoporosis. Unfortunately, many doctors will prescribe medications after a single DXA test, even if the person being tested is under 65. The data that proves pharmaceuticals benefit women under 65 is so lacking that the National Women's Network does not even recommend getting a DXA scan before reaching 65.

Although I applaud the organization's efforts to prevent needless drug treatment, I do not necessarily agree with this position. I feel that having a baseline DXA would allow you and your doctor to assess the velocity of change and how far "up the mountain" you are with bone density. I do, however, agree that DXA results should not be used as a tool to place women on needless pharmaceutical treatment, especially when performed on women under age 65. There is a lot that can be done in the realm of diet, exercise, supplementation, and lifestyle to stabilize and even to improve bone density.

One final note regarding the DXA scan: until the medical community implements a standard for the manufacturer of these scanners, it is important to make sure that your future DXA scans are performed by the same brand of scanner as your previous tests. Researchers have found alarming differences between different scanners that could give inconsistent and inaccurate results. Remember, you cannot rely on your physician to keep tabs on the brand of scanner used, as most of them do not realize that there is a significant difference from brand to brand.

How Much Radiation Does a DXA Scan Expose You to?

The good news is that DXA scans expose you to 3 millirems (mrem) of radiation to evaluate bone density. Allow me to give you a comparison: chest X-rays expose you to 2 to 5 mrem and a coast-to-coast flight exposes you to 5 mrem, almost twice the amount of a DXA scan.

The bottom line is that you have very little to worry about as far as the radiation from a DXA scan is concerned. That being said, radiation exposure is cumulative and thus great care should be taken to limit exposure whenever possible. Except in extreme cases, I can see no reason to get a DXA scan more than every two years.

Why Your DXA Scan May Not Be Accurate

DXA scans are not error-proof—far from it, in fact. Even a technician positioning you incorrectly during the scan can lead to an error in density reading of up to 10 percent. Sadly, many states do not have rules that require special certification for technicians administering the test or even doctors reading the resulting report.

Within radiology, there is a subspecialty called "bone densitometry" that is focused on measurement and interpretation of bone density. An international organization certifies technicians in both the administration and interpretation of tests measuring bone density, yet many states do not require any such certification. This can lead to gross inaccuracies in bone testing that may lead to unnecessary worry and treatment. Improper follow-up tests can also make bone densities appear to be worsening despite stabilization or reversal of bone loss. Technicians and doctors specializing in densitometry are trained to prevent such errors and catch them when they occur, before they can lead to unnecessary drug treatment. It is important to note that one scientific study found that out of 113 DXA scans performed, 61 hips and 94 spines were positioned incorrectly, leading to potentially inaccurate readings (*Clinical Rheumatology,* June 2008).

Every medical test has a margin of error. With the DXA scan, that margin can range between 3 to 5 percent. So, if your result shows a 2 percent change in density from one test to the next, it may not actually mean that you lost or gained 2 percent in bone density; it may just be a standard error caused by variance in the administration of the test. Densitometrists call this variation least significant change (LSC). If a testing center has taken the time, expense, and effort to test their LSC, it will be listed on the test report. If not, you must assume a 3 to 5 percent error. In other words, if the results show a 5 percent loss, you must assume that there was no change in bone density.

Bone Resorption Test – A New Way to Monitor Bone Health NOW!

Bone resorption testing involves a simple urine test that can determine how fast your bones are deteriorating. By testing for collagen crosslinks in the urine—

specifically pyridinium (Pyd) and deoxypyridinium—we can determine how much bone is being broken down. This process is called "bone turnover."

Nearly all women will have a higher rate of bone turnover during the first few years after the onset of menopause (compared to the years prior to menopause). Some women, however, continue to have significantly elevated turnover 10 to 20 years after menopause. Although bone resorption testing does not tell about the density of your bones, it gives important information about whether your body is making deposits or withdrawals from the bone bank account. Therefore, bone resorption testing can be used to evaluate the second piece of the osteoporosis equation regarding bone quality. It can also determine whether supplements and lifestyle changes are working to improve the quality of bones.

This readily available test can give valuable information about how well your bone-building program is working. Simply put, if your bone resorption test result is within the normal range, then at this moment in your life calcium and other important minerals are not being stolen from your precious mineral bank account: the bones. This test is available without a prescription and involves a simple urine collection. Although bone resorption testing indicates nothing about bone density, it speaks to whether your lifestyle is promoting bone wastage or bone growth.

Chapter Summary

People with higher bone density scores experience 63 percent of all fractures (Sheldon, Freemantle et al, University of Leeds: School of Public Health. 1992). Bone quality trumps bone quantity if your goal is to prevent fractures. While a DXA scan does a good job of determining how many minerals are stored up in your skeleton, it does an abysmal job of determining fracture risk. Sadly, there is no readily available bone scan that assesses bone quality. There is an 18-point questionnaire that, although not perfect, may estimate your risk with higher precision than bone density alone. Regardless of your risk, anxiety and worry is not the answer. Your fracture risk can be used to determine how aggressive the bone-building program needs to be. You can reverse bone loss and dramatically improve bone quality through diet, exercise, lifestyle, and supplementation, so keep the faith and read on.

The 18-Point Bone Quality Checklist (It is 18 instead of 17 because I added Proton Pump Inhibitor Use to the list):

1. Do you have poor distance depth perception? (If in doubt, check "yes.")
2. Do you have impaired vision? (Poor vision is a risk factor.)
3. Do you rarely exercise, such as walking or weight lifting? (Sedentary lifestyle is a major risk factor.)
4. Do you have low bone density? (This is *a* risk factor, not *the* risk factor.)
5. Do you take PPIs for reflux or heartburn? (This factor was not in the University of California study but has recently been shown to dramatically increase the risk of fracture.)
6. Do you have trouble getting out of a chair without using your arms? (If you cannot rise from a chair without swinging greatly or using your arms, put a check.)
7. Do you currently use anticonvulsant medications? (These can include

Dilantin®, Neurontin®, Lyrica®, phenytoin, diazepam, etc.)

8. Has your mother had a hip fracture before age 80? (If she has had a fracture, but it occurred after age 80, then leave this blank.)

9. Have you ever been diagnosed with hyperthyroidism? (Hyperthyroidism involves having too much thyroid hormone. Do not confuse this with hypothyroidism, which involves too little thyroid hormone and is not considered a risk factor.)

10. Do you currently use any tranquilizers or mood-altering medications? (This classification includes long-acting benzodiazepines such as alprazolam, chlordiazepoxide, phenobarbital, and any medication that ends in "epam.")

11. Do you have a resting pulse of 80 beats per minute or higher? (Test by checking the pulse in your wrist for 20 seconds and multiplying by 3.)

12. Have you had any fractures since age 50? (This includes any fractures

of a finger, toe, back, hip, etc.)
13. Would you consider yourself in poor health? (Be honest with this question; self-reported poor health is a significant risk factor.)
14. Are you on your feet less than 4 hours per day? (Be honest with this one, too. If you are seated or lying on a couch more than 20 hours a day, then put a check in the box.)
15. Are you a senior citizen? (Sorry, but age does matter, and it does count against you when determining your fracture risk. If you get a discount at restaurants and movie theaters, then answer "yes" to this question.)
16. Do you weigh less today than you did at age 25? (If you weight the same or more than you did at 25, then do not check.)
17. Are you shorter than you were at age 25? (Shrinking is a sign of poor bone quality.)
18. Do you drink caffeinated beverages or use diet pills containing caffeine? (Caffeine causes calcium loss.)

Scoring Your Test

Once you have completed the checklist, add up all the check marks and fill in the number below:

Number of Checks: _____

Good Density/Good Quality

If you scored two checks or fewer *not including low bone density,* then your risk of having an osteoporotic fracture is 1.1 per 1,000 woman-years. This means that your risk of fracture is extremely low due to good density and good quality, Congratulations!

Good Density/Bad Quality

If you scored five checks or more *not including low bone density,* then your risk of having an osteoporotic fracture is 19 per 1,000 woman-years. This means you have normal bone density but poor bone quality. Fracture rates are 19 times higher for women with many of the listed risk factors even though their density may be normal.

Bad Density/Bad Quality

If you scored five checks or more and had low bone density in the osteoporosis range, then your risk of having an osteoporotic fracture is 32 per 1,000 woman-years of life. This group accounts for a full 32 percent of all hip fracture incidences, even though they only account for approximately 6 percent of the female population investigated in this study.

6

Conventional Medicine - Not Always Right, but Never in Doubt

The Missed Boat of Conventional Medicine

Before I get into what I consider to be the most logical, natural approach to the prevention and management—yes, even reversal—of osteoporosis, let us evaluate the conventional medical approach. What you have learned about bones thus far are known biological facts, which, of course, are understood by traditional medicine as well. Conventional medicine took the wrong path, however, when they asked, "How can we get the osteoclasts (bone removers) to stop their work?" instead of asking, "How can we get the osteoblasts (bone builders) to get back to work?" An even better question would be, "How do we optimize the balance between bone-removing cells and bone-building cells so as to mimic the balance we enjoy around age 30?" The traditional medical approach focuses on trying to stop the breakdown of bone, through the taking of such drugs as Fosamax and Premarin®. What these medicines may do in the long-run is proliferate old, brittle, weakened bone instead of helping to create new, young, supple, pliable, and strong bone. Is it possible (some might say even probable) that these medicines could actually make the problem worse over time?

Allow me to paint a metaphorical picture to drive home this point. Imagine a mother bird had just hatched three chicks. She peers into their beautiful little birdy eyes and immediately becomes fearful that eagles circling above will swoop down and snatch one of her little ones. In order to prevent this horrible event from happening, she decides to hop up on the ledge of the nest and watch for eagles 24 hours a day. Yes, this action does protect the birdies from harm in the present, but her inaction due to fear of loss is causing her little beauties to slowly starve to death. As with the conventional approach to treating osteoporosis, working so hard to prevent bone from being taken away can lead to bone cells slowly starving from neglect.

Can You Really Reverse Osteoporosis?

The human body's capacity to repair and to regenerate is nothing short of astounding. Researchers have not directly evaluated how much reversal in bone loss can be achieved through a properly balanced nutrition and lifestyle program; however, numerous studies have proven that supplements and exercise can lead to significant, and even dramatic, changes in bone density. Despite what many doctors may tell you, osteoporosis *can* be reversed without the use of drugs. It takes work, and it takes focus, but you *can* make major improvements.

First, let us take a look at the popular medicines used to treat osteoporosis. Then we will talk about recommendations for prevention and treatment, including proper forms and dosages of specific nutrients. By the end of this book, you will have a system that should help you avoid osteoporosis and reverse a significant amount of bone loss if you are at such a stage. Again, osteoporosis is reversible without medications. It takes work, but you *can* do it.

Of the medications to be discussed, the bisphosphonate class is considered to be the most effective by the medical establishment. Generally speaking, a prescription for a bisphosphonate will almost always accompany a diagnosis of osteopenia or osteoporosis. I will dedicate the majority of the discussion to this class of medication because it is the most popular.

Bisphosphonates – The Flagship Drugs

FOSAMAX® (generic: alendronate)

This drug binds to the bone-removing cells and slows them down. The goal is to make the bone removers slower than the sluggish bone builders. This may sound good initially, and it can be good news if you are at risk of breaking a bone tomorrow; but it also means that you are slowly building new bone around old, brittle bone. What will this mean in 10 to 20 years when you have that many years of old, brittle bone accumulated? The answer is that nobody knows. But we do know who the guinea pigs are: us! So what are the downsides to Fosamax?

- Most people have been prescribed the drug for continual use throughout the rest of their lifetime, yet the drug has only been tested for 3- to 4-year periods. (Data is coming to light that supplementation for longer than five to seven years may be unnecessary and potentially counterproductive.)

- At least some of the drug stays in your bones for life even after discontinuation of the medication. You will never be free of the drug.
- Serious damage to the esophagus is possible if not taken per manufacturer's instructions.
- Bisphosphonates can cause serious heart arrhythmias.
- People taking bisphosphonates have reported muscle and joint pain that may continue even after the drug is stopped.
- The drug is very expensive.

In addition, many dental professionals have recently implicated Fosamax as a potential cause of a condition known as osteonecrosis of the jaw, also known as "Fossy-bone." Fossy-bone is characterized by necrosis or rotting of the jawbone after dental procedures or dental trauma. It commonly becomes a chronic condition and requires antibiotics, antibiotic washes, and close supervision; it also may require surgical procedures in more serious cases. Although 95 percent of jaw-rot cases have been caused by more potent bisphosphonates provided intravenously, more and more cases are being seen in people who took long-term bisphosphonate treatment for osteoporosis in pill form. The FDA recently required a black box warning for all bisphosphonates, such as Fosamax and Actonel, in regard to osteonecrosis of the jaw.

Actonel® (generic: risedronate)

This medication, a close relative to Fosamax, is a "me-too" drug that does not appear to hold any significant benefit over the once-weekly Fosamax. In fact, it appears that Actonel may, in fact, be only half as effective at decreasing hip fracture risk, the most worrisome type of fracture.

Boniva® (Ibandronate Sodium)

Boniva is another close relative of Fosamax and requires only once-monthly dosing. As is the case with Actonel, the risks are similar to other bisphosphonate drugs. This medication is also available in an intravenous (IV) treatment, provided once every three months. The studies to date have been inconclusive on its efficacy. An analysis of the data published to date suggests that the medication decreases the risk of hip fracture by 30 percent. Other studies have found no decrease in the risk of hip fracture.

Reclast (generic: zoledronic acid)

Reclast is a new, once-a-year IV bisphosphonate, prescribed for people who cannot tolerate other bisphosphonates. Expect side effects to be equal to or more severe than other bisphosphonates. Reclast appears to offer a similar level of effectiveness when compared with Fosamax.

Didronel (etidronate) & Aredia (pamidronate)

There is insufficient evidence to suggest that these medications will be as effective as Fosamax, Actonel, Boniva, or Reclast. Therefore, I recommend against taking either of these two medications until more evidence is discovered.

If you do decide to take a bisphosphonate, it may be best to stick with the ones with a longer history of use in patient populations, since they are, at least, the devils we know.

A few more notes about the bisphosphonate class of medication: Commercials make the newer medications (Actonel, Boniva, and Reclast) sound safer and/or more effective because they have a more convenient dosing schedule. In my book, "convenience" is their only bragging right. I have found no evidence that suggests one product is safer or more effective. It can be argued that once-monthly dosing will have less potential for causing damage to the esophagus compared with once-weekly dosing, but even one mishap with any of these medications can lead to severe esophageal damage.

How Effective Are These Medications?

In one of the main studies published on Fosamax, researchers tout a 56 percent decrease in the risk of fracture in participants given Fosamax compared with those on a placebo (sugar pill). This sounds like a significant finding—however, a closer evaluation of this study tells a slightly different story: 99.8 percent of the Fosamax treatment group did not suffer a fracture. That sounds wonderful; however, when you look at the group given an inactive placebo, 99.5 percent of them did not suffer a fracture either. That means the actual difference between the groups was a mere 0.3 percent. This equates to a 56 percent decrease in "relative risk," which is an arbitrary number designed to make the results look more significant than they really are. In other words, you would have to treat 81 women for 4.2 years at a cost of over $300,000 in order to prevent one fracture in a single one of the women. That means 80 out of 81 women will gain *no benefit* from the medication. In my opinion, that is hardly worth the risk.

Now, let us talk about those of you who have been diagnosed with osteopenia (pre-osteoporosis). How did those like you fare in the Fosamax study? Well, according to this research, the subgroup with osteopenia suffered an *increase* in fracture risk, rather than a decrease. In fact, there was an 84 percent increase in the risk of hip fracture and a 50 percent increase in the risk of wrist fracture. This is exactly why I think prescribing these medications for women with osteopenia should be labeled malpractice.

In March 2008, a physician's group published 15 disturbing case reports of women who suffered "atypical low-energy fractures" after using Fosamax. This term refers to fractures that occur in strange places for no apparent reason. Someone could be having a relaxing stroll down the street and bones would just break without causation or warning. This type of fracture typically occurs in extremely frail elderly women. This case report, which was published in the *New England Journal of Medicine,* follows two other negative studies on this class of medication, raising serious questions about the safety of bisphosphonates. It makes much more sense to work to build new, healthy, pliable bone rather than to take a pill that is designed to keep around the old, brittle, damaged bone

Studies are usually conducted in ideal settings in which many variables are carefully controlled. Study participants are usually incentivized to be compliant and often reminded to take their medications. In real-life circumstances, however, people are typically far less compliant than the subjects in the studies. The bisphosphonates are inconvenient to take and sometimes cause stomach upset. Besides, people often just do not like taking medications. The figures presented above are assuming near 100 percent compliance. Truthfully, the benefits are typically inflated, since people simply are not as compliant. Is it possible that the number needed to treat is far greater in real life than is presented in the study? I feel that the answer is a resounding "Yes!"

Painful News About Bisphosphonate Medications

The FDA was forced to issue a press release to the general public as well as a notice to manufacturers of this class of medication, informing patients and doctors about a newly recognized complication: severe and debilitating muscle, bone, and joint pain. This pain can occur days, months, or years after starting bisphosphonate medications, such as Fosamax, Boniva, and Actonel. In my practice, I have spoken with a number of women who suffered incapacitating muscle and joint pain after starting this class of medication. Unfortunately, their doctors failed to recognize that the medications were the cause of this disabling side effect. The fact that it is nearly impossible to know when the side effects will show up makes it very difficult to correlate the onset of pain with the use of medications. Just be aware of this side effect should you ever be prescribed any of the above-mentioned medications. Although the

FDA warning went on to state that some people saw complete remission after stopping the medication, many patients reported only partial remission of pain and others continued to have pain even after the medication had been stopped.

This means that some people will live the rest of their lives in pain because their doctors prescribed a medication that really does little to protect bones in the long run (http://www.fda.gov/cder/drug/infopage/bisphosphonates/default.htm).

One Prescription for Esophageal Cancer, Please...

A recent study published in the *British Medical Journal* discovered a link between bisphosphonate drugs and esophageal cancer. During the course of this study, scientists followed 80,000 men and women for an average of seven years. At the study's end, it was discovered that taking even one prescription of these medications increased the risk of cancer of the esophagus by 30 percent. If the participant used the medication continuously for five years, the risk of cancer doubled. Although that sounds like a huge increase, the incidence of esophageal cancer is approximately 1 in 1,000 people who do not take the medication; the incidence increased to 2 in 1,000 in people who took the medication for at least five years. That is technically a doubling of the risk. We know that bisphosphonates are especially inflammatory to the digestive tract. If there were a significant benefit to using bisphosphonates, we might be able to accept this increased risk in the interest of saving the skeleton from a hip fracture. The problem is, there is very little benefit to taking these drugs. As the side effects mount up, the benefit-to-risk ratio becomes smaller and smaller (*BMJ,* September 2010).

So When is it Appropriate to Use This Medication?

In my opinion, there are two situations when the use of bisphosphonates is warranted: First, if you are at risk of breaking a bone tomorrow, meaning that you are in an emergency state of poor bone health. For our purposes, "poor bone health" equates to having a low bone density and having five or more risk factors for osteoporotic fracture. (See the bone-quality questionnaire.)

The second reason to use bisphosphonates is if you have a low bone density that places you in a state of osteoporosis and just will not do what is necessary to rebuild your bones. I know that sounds harsh, but the truth is that there are people who will not take the supplements necessary or not spend the money on nutritional supplements because they cannot see themselves paying more than a $5.00 co-pay for anything that comes in a pill bottle. Some people would rather pop a pill and spend their precious life sipping on sodas and tossing bonbons into their mouths while lying back and watching television. In my professional opinion, these people should say a quick prayer of thanks for such medications as bisphosphonates. I can only hope that you, your family, and friends do not fall into this group, but if any of you do then this may be an appropriate class of medication, since it could give you a few extra years before you are put into a nursing home with a dangerous hip fracture.

Again, I apologize if this sounds cynical, but I have worked with enough people to know that this type of personality accounts for a good percentage of the population. Good thing for these people that these medications exist.

How Long Should I Be on Bisphosphate Medications, Such as Fosamax and Boniva?

A fascinating study published in the *Journal of the American Medical Association* compared fracture rates in two groups of people: one group received Fosamax for 10 years, and the second group received Fosamax for five years followed by a placebo for five years. At the end of the 10-year study, the fracture risk of the two groups was assessed. The results showed that the two groups were no different in the risk of fracture, despite a 2 or 3 percent loss of bone in the group that took Fosamax for five years (as opposed to 10 years). The take-home message is that five years may be a sufficient period to take the medication for those at high risk of fracture. If we were to add an aggressive supplement and exercise program to the drug, then I would bet that we would see a better bone density and lower risk of fracture than in the 10-year Fosamax treatment group.

One problem with double-blind studies is that they want to answer only one question at a time. This approach is good for the progress of medical science and bad for the folks in the study. Lifestyle is hugely important, so helping all study participants live healthier lives in addition to receiving medical treatment should be optimal (*JAMA,*2006 Dec 27;296(24):2968–9).

According to the Mayo Clinic, "Because of this lingering effect, most experts believe it's reasonable for people who are doing well during treatment—those who have not broken any bones and are maintaining bone density—to consider taking a holiday from their bisphosphonate after taking it for five years."

To bottom line this for you, research appears that stopping your bisphosphonate after five years may provide a benefit to fracture risk similar to that of taking the drug for 10 years.

Are Bisphosphonates Sapping Your Energy and Placing Your Health at Risk?

Many years ago, researchers discovered a compound that was so abundant in the body that they appropriately named it "ubiquinone" because it was so ubiquitous. In fact, every living cell in the body requires ubiquinone in order to produce the energy necessary to function. Ubiquinone, also known as coenzyme Q10, is so important that scientists determined that if coenzyme Q10 levels were to drop by 25 percent the organs would become dysfunctional. If coenzyme Q10 levels dropped by 75 percent, the organism would die.

Later, it was discovered that some medications could actually decrease the body's ability to produce coenzyme Q10. The most well-known medication with this catastrophic effect is the class known as statins, which are used to lower cholesterol. By blocking an enzyme called HMG CoA Reductase, this class of medication inhibits the body from producing coenzyme Q10. The potential result is:

- Fatigue
- Muscle pain
- Liver damage
- Nerve damage
- Heart failure

As you can see, any medication that inhibits coenzyme Q10 production can have catastrophic effects on health and vitality. This could explain why many people report muscle and joint pain after starting a bisphosphonate medication. This also could explain the recent observation that bisphosphonates significantly increase the risk of dangerous heart arrhythmia well and apart from the effects they have on the balance of minerals in the blood.

What to Do if You Are Taking a Bisphosphonate.

If you currently take a bisphosphonate medication, you can supplement the body with coenzyme Q10 (softgel form is preferred) to prevent a deficiency. I recommend taking 100 milligrams (mg) twice daily of a product called ubiquinol. It is widely available at local health-food stores and can be considered quite safe. Please note that, although bisphosphonates inhibit coenzyme Q10 production, they likely also inhibit other important compounds. If coenzyme Q10 does not correct any side effects that you may are be suffering; you may want to reconsider the use of the bisphosphonate and discuss your side effects with the prescribing doctor.

As I have mentioned, a heart arrhythmia can be another side effect of bisphosphonate treatment. An arrhythmia occurs when the heart loses its rhythm, ranging from mild (such as a skipped beat) to serious (such as atrial fibrillation) to deadly (such as ventricular fibrillation, or cardiac arrest). Any of these may occur because of the depletion of coenzyme Q10, although it can more likely be attributed to a mineral imbalance caused by the medication. Such minerals as calcium, potassium, and magnesium are very important to the proper functioning of the heart. If blood levels of these minerals swing too much, the result is an electrical malfunction in the cells of the heart, which can be catastrophic, even causing death. Mineral and coenzyme Q10 supplements may help to prevent this side effect, but they are unlikely to completely ward it off.

Other Medications

Although Fosamax and all of its brothers and sisters are considered the gold standard of osteoporosis care, their side effects often limit their use with many people. But for those who cannot take Fosamax, there are a number of older medications from which to choose.

Miacalcin® (generic: calcitonin-salmon)

This hormonal drug has a similar mechanism of action to Fosamax, in that it decreases the activity of bone-removing cells. It is given in the form of a nasal spray and is approximately half as effective as Fosamax in preventing breakdown of old, brittle bone. Users of this drug should expect approximately a 1.5 percent increase in bone density yearly. The potential side effects of long-term use include sinus irritation, nose bleeds, sinus pain, nausea, vomiting, and facial flushing. This medication is not popular due to a fairly high incidence of nasal irritation and its very modest benefit.

Rocaltrol® (generic: calcitriol)

This drug is basically a patented, expensive, potentially toxic form of vitamin D. It works by increasing the absorption of calcium, decreasing the excretion of calcium, and decreasing the levels of PTH (this will be explained in detail later). I do not generally recommend taking this medication because you can achieve all of these benefits through the appropriate use of one important nutrient. We will look at the natural alternative to this drug later.

Premarin® (generic: conjugated estrogen)

Although this drug has fallen out of favor, it used to be one of the most commonly prescribed medicines. The pill contains many different estrogens collected from pregnant horses, only three of which are also found in the human body. You will recall that estrogen is the hormone that controls the birth and activity of bone-removing cells. Premarin slows the breakdown of bone but has not been shown to build bone. So, typical of western medical thought, this drug is made to try to stop the breakdown of bone rather than proliferate the building of new bone. As for side effects, Premarin clearly increases the risk of breast, uterine, and ovarian cancers. Blood clots, edema, headache, hypertension, increased cholesterol, vaginal bleeding, and weight gain are also commonly reported with use. Lastly, in the first year of taking Premarin, you are more likely to have a heart attack than if you were not on the medication.

In my book, this drug should be removed from the market. With the availability of bioidentical hormone replacement therapy (HRT), there should be no place for such toxic compounds as Premarin. Many women can benefit from bioidentical estrogen, if you are currently taking Premarin or are considering hormone replacement, my suggestion would be to search out a physician who is schooled in the use of natural, bioidentical HRT and pay the extra money for a compounded prescription customized to your needs. To find such a physician, I recommend looking up a local compounding pharmacy in the phonebook or on the web and then asking them to recommend a local doctor who prescribes natural/bioidentical HRT. You may also use the American College for Advancement in Medicine atwww.acam.org. They have a database of more holistically minded physicians that you can search by zip code.

Prolia®, Xgeva® (generic: denosumab)

This newer class of medication appears to work by decreasing the number of bone-removing cells (osteoclasts) that are born into the bone. The end result is fewer cells eating up old bone. Whereas bisphosphonate drugs poison existing bone-breaking cells, this class of drugs prevents them from being born in the first place. These medications are usually used as a bisphosphonate alternative for people who cannot take such drugs as Fosamax due to kidney issues or digestive problems. They appear to provide a small benefit to fracture risk but, like bisphosphonates, will likely lead to poor quality bone over time, only slowing the removal of old bone.

Forteo® (generic: teriparatide) and Tymlos (generic: abaloparatide)

These are the only drugs that possibly can increase bone remodeling (bone formation). Due to the potential for severe side effects, these drugs are usually reserved for certain high-risk populations, such as those who have suffered osteoporotic fractures and/or bone loss due to steroid use. Sadly, these drugs can cause a dangerous elevation in blood calcium levels that can affect the heart.

True Story

Lori is a 50-year-old, post-menopausal woman who goes to her doctor annually for a checkup. Her doctor orders a DXA scan in order to get a baseline value for comparison in later years. The DXA comes back in the normal range with no indication of osteopeniaor osteoporosis. On the next visit, the doctor writes a prescription for Fosamax and explains to Lori that although her bone density is fine, the doctor does not want her to begin a downward turn that would be expected at the onset of menopause.

I submit this ridiculous-but-true case because it is a prime example of the American medical system's philosophy that it is okay to die with medications but it is not okay to die without medications. There is absolutely no proof that the benefits of Fosamax or any bisphosphonate medication would outweigh the negative effects of this class of medication. In fact, common sense and current evidence would suggests that this type of prescribing practice would place this woman of just 50 years at a significant risk of fracture and Fossy-bone in her golden years. A ridiculous prescription that, in my book, borders on malpractice.

Chapter Summary:

Most medications prescribed to treat osteoporosis work by inhibiting the cells responsible for cleaning old, brittle bone from the body. Therefore, most medications do little to build bone and lead instead to the accumulation of poor-quality bone over time. Clearly, a better approach is needed if the goal is to build resilient bones. Remember, bone density is only one factor that can contribute to bone strength. You can have lots of bone and still suffer a fracture because the quality of the bone is subpar. Most drugs may artificially raise bone density while simultaneously decreasing bone quality.

7

Hormones The Heal, Hormones That Steal

PTH – The Robin Hood of Bones

PTH monitors and adjusts calcium levels in the blood. Calcium is needed for the proper function of the heart, muscles, cells, and bones. The skeleton is the body's bank account for calcium and many other minerals. When there is not enough calcium floating around in the bloodstream for use by the body, then PTH goes to the bank and makes a withdrawal. In a sense, it steals from the calcium rich (bones) and gives to the calcium poor (blood). This process is designed to be a lifesaving measure. Lack of calcium in the blood can be responsible for heart rhythm irregularities, possibly leading to death. However, when your blood calcium levels are chronically low, PTH is working overtime. This is one of the reasons why osteoporosis is so prevalent in this country. Many practitioners believe that overproduction of PTH is a significant cause of osteoporosis, osteoarthritis, bone spurs, calcium deposits in the arteries (arteriosclerosis), and mental decline. But what would lead to an elevation in parathyroid levels?

Because our bodies were specifically designed to function amidst famine, we have backup mechanisms that retain the critically important processes to avoid acute dangers to our health. So, even though maintaining blood calcium levels by stealing minerals from bones can eventually lead to osteoporosis, it is a sacrifice the human body's inherent intelligence is willing to make in order to prevent your heart from stopping or vital organs from shutting down in the immediate future.

During a famine, your mineral intake may be significantly lower than is necessary to maintain body processes. In this situation, the body must make a withdrawal from the mineral bank account (bones). PTH is the hormone that is charged with the dirty deed of robbing the bone bank account. Ideally, PTH elevates and then quickly returns to normal. Such pulses of PTH actually have a positive impact on bones due to a feedback system that ultimately triggers bones to grab and to store more minerals to prepare the body for the next famine. However, when PTH is chronically elevated, there is no such benefit. In fact, bones are constantly being robbed of these vital minerals, and osteoporosis ensues.

Any natural program that stimulates the strengthening of bones needs to control the PTH levels as a primary or secondary mechanism of action. If this does not occur, then it will be nearly impossible to improve the strength and quality of bone. It is the proverbial "one step forward, two steps back." We will discuss this in detail throughout the book as many approaches that have a positive influence on bone resilience help to normalize PTH levels. This section just sets the stage for the discussion by providing a fundamental understanding of this important hormone.

The Truth About Sex Hormones (Estrogen, Progesterone, etc.)

Estrogen is the hormone that you most commonly hear about whenever the discussion of osteoporosis comes up. If we look at estrogen from the standpoint of evolution, estrogen plays a critically important role in conserving calcium so that the mother can provide milk to nourish her growing child. This process, of course, requires high levels of calcium.

Estrogen appears to partially accomplish this conservation effect by inhibiting PTH, increasing the absorption of calcium, and decreasing the loss of calcium from the bones. Note that estrogen's main role is not to grow bone but to conserve calcium and bone by inhibiting the activity of the bone removers (osteoclasts).

Progesterone is an ovarian hormone that plays a much more important role in the growth of bone. Osteoblasts, the bone-building cells, contain receptors for progesterone, which stimulates them to do their job. Research involving young female athletes has found that these women, who have abnormal menstrual periods due to excessively low progesterone levels, can have significantly lower bone densities compared with athletes with normal progesterone secretion. In fact, it is common to see up to 3 percent decreases in bone density per year of abnormal menstruation in young women (*JAMA,* 263.4;1990: 545–548). This same progesterone disturbance occurs in women as they approach menopause, when the menstrual cycle naturally becomes abnormal. In fact, research has found that bone loss during the perimenopausal time can occur at a much faster rate than the postmenopausal period. Supplementation with natural progesterone has shown to be clinically effective at helping to reverse bone loss. Never forget that progesterone is just one factor in the process of bone remodeling.

Also, remember that all progesterone medications are not created equal. Medroxyprogesterone, the most commonly prescribed form of progesterone-like compounds, is a synthetic progesterone mimic. This means it is not identical to your body's own progesterone—and the body is not fooled. Medroxyprogesterone is 35 times stronger than natural, bioidentical progesterone and has been linked to a higher incidence of breast cancer, heart disease, and stroke. According to Robert Langer, MD, MPH, professor of family and preventative medicine at the University of California, San Diego, School of Medicine, natural progesterone results in fewer days of bleeding and less intense bleeding than the progesterone mimics (*Bottom Line's Health Breakthroughs,* 2004). Micronized progesterone is available over the counter in a topical cream and as a prescription in capsule form. Seek out a medical professional with experience in natural HRT to have a customized hormone plan designed for your unique system.

What About Surgically Induced Menopause?

Every year, over 500,000 women undergo surgical procedures to remove their ovaries, sending them into surgically induced menopause. The majority will begin to show signs of osteoporosis within four years of surgery. These women should investigate natural/bioidentical HRT in order to prevent this osteoporotic fate. For anyone who was prescribed Premarin or Prempro®, you would do yourself a great service by finding a physician trained in bioidentical HRT. Because these hormones are derived from pregnant horses, they contain a number of estrogens that are naturally found only in horses, which have much more potent effects in women and are likely culprits in increasing the risk of various cancers. Bioidentical HRT attempts to mimic the body's secretion of hormones that are chemically identical to the hormones produced by the human body. A properly prescribed and monitored bioidentical hormone replacement program can limit risk and optimize benefits.

What If I Had A Partial Hysterectomy That Left The Ovaries Intact?

This is a common question—and one for which there is a lot of misinformation. Theoretically, leaving the ovaries should prevent the need for supplementation with natural progesterone. The problem is, up to half of women who have an ovary-sparing hysterectomy will have ovarian failure, in which the "spared" ovaries becoming phantom organs that do not produce significant levels of hormones. Women who have a partial hysterectomy still need to follow up with a physician schooled in bioidentical hormones in order to evaluate their need for progesterone and estrogen replacement (*Fertil Steril.* 47.1; 1987: 94–100).

What About Men?

Men can also have hormonal deficiencies that result in an increased likelihood of osteoporosis. This can start in adolescence if the onset of puberty was later than age 13.5 because their bone may never reach its peak mass (*N Engl J Med.* 1992:326.9:600–604). In addition, having a vasectomy may increase your risk of developing osteoporosis later in life due to the altered production of testosterone. Men should have their testosterone levels assessed to evaluate the need for testosterone replacement therapy. This is especially the case if men have an unexpected change in bone density not caused by certain medications, such as antacids, PPIs, and steroids (prednisone). Women may also benefit from the bone-building benefit of testosterone if they show lower than optimal levels for their gender.

Chapter Summary

Chronically elevated parathyroid hormone is a significant cause of osteoporosis. If your intake of minerals is insufficient, this can lead to a slow erosion of bone due to this elevation in parathyroid hormone. Estrogen, progesterone, and testosterone can all be allies in the fight against osteoporosis. You should consider seeking the advice of a physician who is trained in the use of bioidentical HRT to determine if this is a viable tool for you and your circumstances.

8

The Bone Resiliency Formula

Earlier, I introduced you to Dr. Brown's formula for bone fracture risk:

Thin Osteoporotic Bone (Low Density) + Poor Bone Self-Repair = Bone Fracture Risk

It does a pretty good job of uncovering a new model for how bones get weaker despite medicine's best efforts. In this chapter, we will build upon this work and introduce you to the formula for resilient bones.

Resilient Bones Is the Goal

The world seems to be obsessed with bone density—but density, as it turns out, is a poor indicator of how likely your bones are to fracture. Moving forward, it is better to think in terms of bone resiliency over bone density. It is true that there is a correlation between the two; generally speaking, resilient bones will present as denser bones. Sadly, the opposite is not true; density tells us very little about bone resiliency.

Confused? I can liken the distinction between resiliency and density to the process of losing weight. Let us say that you want to lose weight; I can help you achieve your weight-loss goals by locking you in a dungeon and not feeding you for a month, or I can teach you to eat a nutritious diet and exercise regularly. Both will result in significant amounts of weight loss, however, one approach will result in a "skin and bones" version of yourself, while the other will have you looking strong, energetic, and healthy. That is density versus resiliency. Taking a drug that increases density at the expense of bone quality is equivalent to weight loss via the "Dungeon Diet."

Bone resilience is defined as resistance to fractures during physical challenges of everyday life. You should be able to walk, jog, and run with confidence that you are not going to spontaneously fracture a bone. You should be able to tolerate a fall, consistent with daily life challenges, without fracturing a bone. We are not talking about out-of-the-ordinary traumatic events, such as falling from a high ladder or being in a bad car accident. Ideally, your bones should be able to withstand a physical trauma of daily living that a 30- to 40-year-old person could withstand without fracturing a bone. That is bone resilience.

In my work, I have met senior women who have low bone density and high bone resilience. How do we know? They report falling hard but being able to get up and walk it off without a fracture. My own mother, at age 81, went sliding into third base at her retirement community softball game without more than a scratch or two. Bone resiliency is all that matters. Everything else is information, not destiny. Loss of bone density—i.e., decreases in mineralization of the bone— is a sign that bone quality is also being eroded. Simply stated, resilient bones do not generally lose minerals. That being said, loss of bone density is not a guarantee that bones are prone to fracture. As I reported earlier, architecturally speaking the bone structure could theoretically lose up to 50 percent of its structure and still be able to withstand significant amounts of stress without fracture. That is if the bone that is present is resilient.

How Do You Measure Bone Resilience?

Sadly, there currently is no good measure of bone resiliency. We cannot scan your bones or give you a blood test to determine the fracture resistance of your bones. The best measure of bone resiliency is the questionnaire provided in the previous chapter. That being said, that is where the Bone Resiliency Formula comes into play.

The Bone Resiliency Formula:

(Building Blocks X Osteogenic Stimulation) - Resistance Factors = Bone Resilience

Let's take each component of this formula to learn how we can use it to build a plan forward.

Resiliency Factor #1: Building Blocks

You cannot build a house without the right building blocks. Similarly, you cannot build bones without the right building blocks. If you are deficient in one or more core building blocks, then your bone resilience will suffer. There are three core building blocks, which we will cover in future chapters: vitamins, minerals, and collagen peptides. Imagine building a house without wood or nails or plaster. That is similar to attempting to build bones when a component is missing. Your body will do its best with the resources available to it, but it will not be able to build an optimal structure without all of the needed building blocks.

Resiliency Factor #2: Osteogenic Stimulation

If you have plenty of building material but the workers are all sleeping on the job, the house will never get built. Even if a few workers do manage to get to work, you can bet the house will not be built well. Similarly, if you have lots of minerals, vitamins, and protein floating through the blood but the bone builders are dormant or absent, your bone resiliency will suffer greatly.

This explains why the national recommendation to push calcium down the throats of seniors has been notoriously ineffective at preventing osteoporosis in our country. We are delivering lots of wood to a worksite, yet the workers are asleep or absent. To improve the resiliency of bone, we must do more than simply slow bone loss; we must stimulate the bone-building cells to get to work laying down new bone using the wonderful building blocks that we are sending into the bloodstream. How do we achieve this goal?

Osteoblasts are notoriously difficult to activate using drugs and chemicals, which is why drug companies have focused on poisoning the bone-removing cells rather than activating the bone builders. Certain vitamins, such as vitamin K (more on this later), can nudge the bone builders into action. However, there is only one method that is *proven* to trigger the bone-building cells to get into massive action laying down resilient bone characterized by density, strength, and pliability. The method is called "osteogenic loading."

I am going to go out on a limb and predict that if you were to line up 20 senior citizens, I could determine with far better accuracy than a DXA scanner who would make it the next 10 years or so without fractures. How? I would test their physical strength. Generally, the stronger the person, the stronger the bones because when the body is forced to carry heavier loads, the body responds by building stronger bones.

Osteogenic stimulation is defined as exposing the skeleton to a sufficient load to trigger the bone remodeling process (bone strengthening).

The Law Of Need - The Reason Why Osteogenic Stimulation Is The Lynchpin

The Law of Need states that bones are as strong as they *need* to be. Assuming that you have sufficient building blocks and are not exposed to resistance factors (discussed in the next section), then your bones will be sufficiently strong to handle the stresses placed upon them.

The reason this law is so vitally important to our plan moving forward is that it explains why drugs and supplements used as sole strategies for preventing osteoporosis fail to deliver results beyond slowing bone loss in many people.

Drugs alone violate this law. Supplements alone violate this law.

The best place we see the Law of Need in action is in astronauts who return from extended stays in space, their bodies riddled with osteoporosis from weeks or months of zero gravity. Likewise, a similar phenomenon occurs in people on bed rest (what researchers call microgravity); within months they can become osteoporotic. A body on bed rest does not need strong bones, and so the bones lose strength, density, and resilience.

If you are sedentary, your bones are as strong as they need to be to carry your body weight and no stronger.

Osteoporotic fractures occur in moments of challenge beyond your normal body weight, such as falls, accidents, or trauma beyond the normal everyday load that your body is acclimated to handle. The problem is, in the moments that you *need* strong bones, they are not available.

An ounce of prevention is worth a gallon of treatment. If you are strong beyond your age, then you likely have bones that are also stronger than the average of someone in your age group. Why? The loads that have been placed upon your body over the years have sent signals that you need more bone to handle those loads. Those signals have slowed or prevented the bone loss that normally occurs with age, as people naturally lose strength and muscle.

Okay, so you have lost muscle/strength. What now?

I have good news and bad news: The good news is that you *can* reverse bone loss by building muscular strength—in essence, using the Law of Need to your advantage. The bad news is that research suggests you must expose the body to four times your body weight to trigger what is called an osteogenic load. In other words, if you weigh 120 pounds, you need to lift 480 pounds to trigger the hip and leg bones to start growing more dense and resilient. That may be a depressing thought, since many people tell me they can barely lift a milk jug much less 480 pounds. Do not worry. I will get into safe ways to trigger osteogenic load in the body in a future chapter. For now, just know that taking measures to build physical strength will help you build stronger bones through the second resilience factor: osteogenic stimulation.

Resilience Factor #3 - Resistance Factors

Resistance factors are the only component of the formula that works against bone resilience. We want fewer resistance factors in our lives if our goal is to build resilient bones. A resistance factor is anything that we expose ourselves to voluntarily or involuntarily that erodes our skeleton and opposes our bone resilience. Sadly, there are many factors that can work against our efforts to build and to maintain healthy bones.

Here is a list of common resistance factors that work against your bones and can lead to secondary osteoporosis:

1. PPIs for GERD
2. Antidepressants
3. Steroid medications (prednisone, prednisolone, etc.)
4. Thyroid medications
5. Celiac disease
6. Crohn's disease
7. Chronic stress
8. Elevated homocysteine
9. Untreated hyperthyroidism
10. Smoking
11. Alcohol abuse
12. Kidney failure
13. Anorexia/eating disorders
14. Rheumatoid arthritis
15. COPD
16. Multiple sclerosis

17. Diabetes
18. Lithium
19. Hyperparathyorid

The more resistance factors that you tolerate in your life, the more difficult it will be to prevent and/or reverse bone loss. Some resistance factors are out of your control, but that does not mean all hope is lost. Using the Bone Resilience Formula, you can counteract the negative effects of resistance factors by assuring you have the needed building blocks and by pursuing an aggressive plan to trigger an osteogenic load.

The Bone Resilience Formula may be the most important lesson in this book. The more you make use of this formula to improve your lifestyle, the more success you will have in building fracture-resistant bones. In the coming chapters, we will discuss specific ways to use this formula for the benefit of your skeleton.

Chapter Summary:

The Bone Resiliency Formula is a simple approach to improving bone density. By delivering the proper building blocks, activating bone builder cells through osteogenic stimulation, and by limiting the resistance factors that work to erode your bones you can build stronger bones.

9

The Calcium Controversy

GOT MILK? Still Got Osteoporosis

Milk has calcium ... calcium is needed for bones ... therefore, milk *must* prevent osteoporosis ... right? Wrong! This myth has been disproved in numerous studies, including the Harvard Nurses' Health Study. This study of 75,000 nurses over 12 years found that dairy did not protect the nurses from osteoporosis, and the milk drinkers were even shown to have a higher risk of fractures (*Am J Public Health* 1997; 87: 992–7). This negative finding was confirmed by another study published in the *New England Journal of Medicine.* In this study, researchers found no correlation between dairy intake and a lesser risk of hip fractures (*N Engl J Med.* 1995: 332: 767–73). I am sorry for resorting to a listing of research, but people will not otherwise accept that dairy is not a healthy food for bones. As recently as August 2009, researchers suggested that young adults are not drinking enough milk even though the focus of the study was on calcium intake. All too often, dairy is promoted as the sole source of calcium rather than one source of many. It is easy to interpret a study on dietary calcium intake as a study promoting the benefits of dairy despite the fact that calcium can come from other, non-dairy sources.

We are going to stick by the adage that dairy is food for baby cows but not for humans. We are not only the sole species to drink milk past infancy, but also the only species to drink the milk of another animal. Remember that our country has among the highest dairy intake and still has among the highest incidence of osteoporosis.

But Is Milk Not the Best Source of Calcium?

It is true that milk is a source of calcium. It is not true, however, that milk is the best absorbed and utilized form of calcium. One study found that the calcium found in milk has a modest absorption of approximately 32 percent. This means that if you drank enough milk to provide 1,000 mg of calcium, then you would only absorb 320 mg. That same study discovered that calcium from vegetables can be far better absorbed; in fact, it is estimated that 40 to 64 percent of the calcium in vegetables will be absorbed. That means for every 1,000 mg of calcium that you consume from vegetable sources you will absorb between 400 to 640 mg (*Am J Clin Nut*, April 1990; 51, 656–657).

Did you know that scientists estimate that bone-building minerals and nutrients in fruits and vegetables have decreased by over 40 percent since 1940? Another report published in 1992 reported that the mineral content of American soil had decreased by 85 percent. Poor-quality soil results in poor-quality fruits and vegetables; after all, without minerals the plants cannot produce vitamins. This decrease has occurred due to poor farming practices, such as the use of less nutritive fertilizers, poor crop rotation, the use of dams, and overfarming of land. In addition, many of the fruits and vegetables are picked at an unripe stage and then artificially ripened on the way to the consumer. A 1999 report out of Rutgers University determined that conventional fruits and vegetables contained just 16 percent of the minerals found in organic, vine-ripened equivalents. All of these factors culminate in fruits and vegetables that are less nutritive, which is why everybody should take part in some degree of supplementation to act as an insurance policy against rogue deficiency that can cause your bones to weaken.

One final note for the skeptics out there: did you know that calorie for calorie, turnip greens have three times more calcium than milk?

Calcium – Everything You Need to Know

It is a common myth that calcium is the only mineral that bones need to grow. We have been preaching for years the importance of a bone mineral formula in building strong, healthy, pliable bones. Taking calcium alone to build bones is like trying to build a house with only wood. Could you build a house without also using nails, plaster, plastic, glass, etc.? Of course not! So why would you believe that you could build bones, a structure much more complex than a house, by just adding calcium?

The fact is, your bones are not made up of calcium alone, but also magnesium, strontium, silica, boron, other minerals, and protein. Look to later sections to describe the importance of these other minerals, but, for now, let us get into the various forms of calcium. These days many of our foods are "fortified" with calcium, so why are we still deficient?

There are several reasons for this.

Calcium Carbonate (Oyster Shell, Tums®, Viactiv®, Oscal®)

When was the last time you ate an oyster shell? We should not have to say more, but we will. Calcium carbonate is a cheap form of calcium derived from the oyster shell. The irony here is that the oyster shell was designed by nature and millions of years of evolution to prevent the ingestion of the animal inside. Yet after we eat the animal inside, crush up the shell (because we would never be able to chew and swallow the shell as it comes), and make it into a tablet, it becomes the most popular and least effective osteoporosis solution known to man. In order to absorb the calcium from the oyster shell, we must have sufficient acid in the stomach. However, calcium carbonate is, itself, an antacid—and there goes the logic.

Does calcium carbonate get absorbed? The answer is yes. However, the absorption is clearly less than other forms of calcium, especially in certain populations. Senior citizens already produce less hydrochloric acid in their stomachs. In this population, calcium carbonate has a whopping 5 percent absorption (*Nutrition Reviews.* 52: 221, 1994). Additionally, with the abuse of such drugs as Prilosec®, Prevacid®, Tagamet®, Pepcid®, and Zantac® (all work to decrease acid production), many younger people are now living with the digestive abilities of the typical 90 year old. With the combination of these drugs and the antacid properties of the calcium carbonate, the absorption is almost nil. If you have calcium carbonate in your medicine cabinet, just toss it in the trash.

Calcium Citrate (Citrical)

Calcium citrate is a readily absorbable and inexpensive form of calcium. Unlike calcium carbonate, it does not require an acidic stomach to be absorbed. Even when stomach acid is low, 40 to 45 percent of the calcium in calcium citrate gets absorbed. This result was produced under the same conditions under which calcium carbonate showed a mere 5 percent acceptable absorption (*Nutrition*

Review. 52: 221, 1994). If cost is the chief consideration, this form of calcium may offer the best option for the price. Remember that calcium alone, in any form, is still just one piece of the puzzle. A bothersome issue about calcium citrate is the fact that this form of calcium may significantly increase the absorption of lead and aluminum in the diet (*Southern Med J,* 87 (9): 894–8). It is not yet known if this is clinically significant, but I feel that calcium citrate is a safe and effective form of calcium, with a cost that is only modestly more expensive than calcium carbonate.

Calcium Citrate-Malate

This form of calcium combines calcium citrate and calcium malate, usually in equal amounts. The final product seems to enhance the solubility and bioavailability of the calcium. This form is probably superior to calcium citrate alone; however, therapeutically the difference may be minimal. If available, I recommend using this form over standard citrate, but I would not worry if calcium citrate is all that is available to you. A side benefit of the "malate" in this formula is that it can be shuttled into the cell and used to energize it.

Microcrystalline Hydroxyapatite (MCHA)

This is one of our favorite sources of calcium because it best matches the form found in human bones. MCHA (the fancy scientific name for this bone meal) is a wonderful matrix of calcium, phosphorus, and proteins that occur naturally in bone in the right proportions to stimulate bone formation. In a study comparing calcium gluconate with MCHA, the group receiving no mineral supplement showed progressive bone loss, the calcium gluconate group had no significant change in bone density, and the MCHA group had significant gains in bone density. In all groups, vitamin D was given (*Amer J Clin Nutrition.* 36, 426–430; 1982). Another study of 25 osteoporotic patients found virtually no change in the MCHA group, while the control group lost 5.8 percent of total bone density (*New England Journal of Medicine.* 316(4):173–177). In an editorial published in a well-respected medical journal, a researcher endorsed MCHA as the preferred source of calcium over calcium carbonate and gluconate, describing calcium carbonate as "interfering with digestion" (*British Medical Journal,* 2(6145):1124). To date, MCHA is the only form of calcium to show benefit to both trabecular bone (the soft inner core of bone tissue) and cortical bone (the hard outer layer) (*Amer J Clin Nutrition.* 36, 426–430; 1982; *J. Royal Soc. of Medicine.*73:780–85).

This form of calcium is, of course, not appropriate for vegetarians. I suggest any of the other forms of calcium with the exception of calcium carbonate.

Calcium Amino Acid Chelates

When calcium is bound to amino acids (building blocks of protein), it becomes an organic calcium compound. The body then absorbs the amino acid through the intestinal wall and carries it with the calcium into the bloodstream, where cells take in the amino acid and calcium. As the amino acid is metabolized, the calcium is liberated so that cells can utilize it. This is one of the key ways to get minerals into cells where they can be efficiently used. It is nature's preferred way of mineral delivery and similar to the calcium found in the vegetables we eat. Chelated calcium can be difficult to find, and I wouldn't spend too much time trying to find a formula that uses this type of calcium, as most other forms will suffice.

So What Does All This Mean? What Type, How Much, and When?

Each person seems to respond differently to the various forms of calcium. Some people prefer capsules, others prefer tabs, and some prefer liquid. There is still a lot of debate over which is the best form of calcium and how much is the most effective dose. I believe that the chelated form of calcium and MCHA are best, as they mimic the types of calcium found in food. I have used the MCHA form of calcium with good results in my practice. The government suggests a dose of 1,200 to 1,500 mg of calcium daily; keep in mind, however, that this amount is the total from food and supplements. Many doctors erroneously recommend that their patients take 1,200 to 1,500 mg of calcium in supplements without realizing that the average person gets 600 to 800 mg of calcium from their diet.

We suggest just 500 to 800 mg of calcium in supplement form and no more. This should be plenty for the body as long as you take one of the above-mentioned forms of calcium and balance it with magnesium and other nutrients. Some experts suggest calcium be taken at night to help prevent the surge in PTH that is believed to rob bones of calcium during slumber. I see nothing wrong with this philosophy but feel that it is likely splitting hairs and unlikely to make a significant difference.

If 500 to 800 mg of Calcium is Good; Will 1200 to 1500 mg Not Be Better?

The answer is no. The belief that calcium alone is sufficient to keep bones healthy is a fallacy. In fact, recent research suggests that the calcium needs of the human body have been grossly overestimated. In fact, it is now estimated that the body needs just 750 mg of calcium daily to be in balance, instead of the 1,200 to 1,500 mg estimates of yesteryear (*American Journal of Clinical Nutrition.* 86(4):1054–63). There *is* such a thing as too much of a good thing when discussing nutrition and supplementation. It is important that you not overload your body with excess levels of any particular nutrient, as this could throw other nutrients out of balance (such as magnesium, zinc, and iron). In fact, some preliminary research suggests that people who have excessive intakes of calcium could increase the risk of calcification of the arteries, heart disease, and stroke (*British Medical Journal.* 336

(7638):262–266). Other data has contradicted the research that suggests calcium increases the risk of calcified arteries; however, I feel it wise not to overload the body with any vitamin or mineral. Remember, the body seeks balance; taking large quantities of calcium throws off that delicate balance.

I also hypothesize that calcium (and other minerals) may be more effective in smaller doses if those amounts are taken throughout the day with meals. For example, I suspect that taking 100 mg of calcium three times daily may be more effective than taking 300 mg of calcium twice daily. Right now, it is just a hypothesis, but if you are concerned about calcium causing problems with your arteries, take a smaller dose more often throughout the day as an alternative to larger doses at fewer times.

Reasons For Deficiency

I am often asked why anyone would be deficient in calcium. The answer is probably multifactorial. We already discussed that the soil is depleted, which leads to fewer minerals per pound of fruits and vegetables that we consume. Aside from the depleted nutritive value of those fruits and vegetables available to us, we also eat far fewer of them.

In addition to the poor quality of the food we consume, our digestive tracts are in disarray, with many people suffering from low stomach acid from lifestyle, age, and such antacid drugs as Tums®, Mylanta®, Maalox®, Zantac®, Prilosec®, Tagamet®, and Nexium®. Low stomach acid makes it difficult to liberate the already deficient minerals from the food, resulting in poor intake and poor absorption of minerals and vitamins. Vitamin D deficiency, epidemic in our society, further interferes with the absorption of the few minerals we eat and liberate from food.

These are just a few on the mounting list of resistance factors that work against our bones and set us up for deficiencies of these vital minerals.

What if Calcium Constipates Me?

This is a fairly common issue for people who are supplementing with calcium. There are a number of things that can be successfully done to remedy this issue.

Keep well hydrated: If you are even mildly dehydrated, then the stool will dry up and literally act as a plug in the colon. Calcium-induced constipation is worsened when the bowels are dry.

Balance calcium intake with magnesium intake: Magnesium can help keep the fluid balanced in the intestines, thus preventing the drying of the stool. Constipation most commonly occurs in people who dose high in calcium with little or no magnesium. If constipation is a problem, I recommend finding a product that uses a ratio of calcium to magnesium closer to 1:1 (1 mg of magnesium for each 1 mg of calcium) or simply adding more magnesium to balance the calcium.

Vitamin D: If your body is unable to absorb minerals into the bloodstream, then more will be retained in the colon to cause constipation. By taking an appropriate dose of vitamin D, you can enhance your mineral absorption. (We will discuss vitamin D in detail in the forthcoming section.)

Cut the dose of calcium: Many people are simply taking too much calcium and may be especially sensitive to even small amounts of calcium. Most people require only 600 to 800 mg of calcium balanced with 300 to 800 mg of magnesium. If you are inclined to have calcium-induced constipation, then you may be able to take only 200 to 300 mg of calcium. Not to worry, this does not mean you are going to develop osteoporosis.

If all else fails, try a formula called 3A Magnesia by Lane Medical. This specially processed magnesium formula significantly increases lubrication in the bowels and stimulates motility. I suggest two to four tablets at night before bedtime, increasing to six tabs for one or two nights in stubborn cases. Customize the dose to your response. If you are taking other sources of magnesium, then you may require only one or two tablets. Play with the dose until you find what works for you. Please note that this form of magnesium is designed to improve bowel function; it does not replace the magnesium used to treat osteoporosis because it is made to *not* be absorbed into the bloodstream. Rather, it stays in the bowel.

What Happens if I Just Cannot Take Any Calcium without Getting Severe Constipation or Digestive Upset?

Simple, do not take calcium.

But do not fret: you can support your bones through the optimization of vitamin D to enhance your absorption of calcium through diet and add many other vital nutrients and minerals that will support bone health. You can also increase your dietary intake of foods high in calcium, such as green, leafy vegetables; fruits; and nuts. Many foods are fortified with additional calcium, and thus you are likely getting 600 to 800 mg of calcium daily anyway, which appears to be sufficient to meet the needs of the body.

Newer food-sourced mineral formulas may provide a "gentler" experience for you because the minerals are in the food matrix form. For a list of supplement recommendations, visit OsteoCoach.com/StrongBonesForever.

Constipation can be a serious problem for many people, especially as they age. I believe that no nutritional formula should be used if it causes negative side effects. Nutrition should result in you feeling better, not worse. Unlike medications, nutrition should come free of side effects; if side effects are noted, simply alter the program or stop the product altogether.

Should Calcium and Magnesium Be Taken Separately?

I have heard some authors and experts claim that calcium and magnesium compete for absorption. They then recommend separating the two supplements in order to enhance absorption. I do not recommend this for two reasons:

Life is complicated enough. I try to keep the supplement programs as simple as possible.

Nature provides minerals together. Show me an example in nature where a food source contains only one mineral. There are none. Mother Nature is not worried about mineral competition, and neither am I.

What If I Can't Swallow Pills?

Please do not opt for the tasty little calcium chews as the majority of these products use calcium carbonate. Good sources of calcium are available in many forms, including liquid and chewable tablets. Please refer to the resource list for specific brands and products at OsteoCoach.com/StrongBonesForever.

Could Your Osteoporosis Be a Sign of Stomach Acid Deficiency?

Conventional medicine seems to believe that proper digestion is unnecessary for health. Walking into the doctor's office with any kind of digestive complaint almost guarantees that you will walk out with a prescription for some sort of antacid medication. This is a disturbing practice because many of these medications have been linked to osteoporosis. The fact is, nature put acid in your stomach for many very important reasons. One such reason is to ionize minerals so that they can be absorbed into the bloodstream.

Many factors interfere with digestion:
- Stress
- Medications
- Calcium carbonate (Tums, Viactive®, OsCal®, etc.)
- Age

With poor digestion an epidemic in our society, many doctors now believe that can be to blame for many osteoporosis cases. Do everything that you can to avoid having to use antacid medications. If you have digestive problems, seek out an integrative physician who can help you to resolve these issues.

Contrary to popular belief, heartburn/GERD is not caused by too much acid in a great majority of people. Rather, it is usually due to a failure of the esophageal sphincter, the doorway between the stomach and the esophagus. The result is stomach contents refluxing back into the esophagus and thus irritating its delicate lining. Even low stomach acid is acidic enough to irritate and damage the esophageal lining. When you eat, stomach acid begins to rise, which tells the body that you are digesting food. In a healthy body, the rising acid triggers the body to close the esophageal sphincter, which keeps the contents of the stomach sequestered during digestion. If you suffer from low stomach acid, the doorway between the stomach and esophagus does not get the signal that you are digesting food and thus does not close. This results in the contents of the stomach refluxing up into the esophagus where it causes damage. The cause of most reflux then is low stomach acid, rather than excess stomach acid.

Although the proper treatment of GERD is beyond the scope of this book, I can recommend *Natural Solutions for Digestive Health* by Jillian Teta, ND.

Getting the Lead Out

In recent years, there have been concerns about the lead content of calcium supplements. In a study published in April 2000, researchers tested 136 leading brands of calcium supplements and found that two-thirds of the brands did not meet the California criteria for acceptable lead content (*Environ Health Perspec,* April 2000; 108(4): 309–313). For this reason it is important to choose quality brands that regularly test their finished products for lead levels.

It is impossible to remove 100 percent of the lead from calcium supplements, although as stated above you can minimize the intake of lead from these sources. The lead content in the diet is estimated to be 5 to 11 micrograms (mcg) per day; however, these levels are very dynamic. Simply adding a glass of wine to the diet can increase the daily intake of lead to 75 mcg (*Chem Spec & Bioavail.* 3, 31–36). The FDA Total Diet Study 1991–93 found the following levels of lead in dairy sources (per 1,000 mg of calcium):

- Whole milk: 1.68 to 6.72 mcg
- 2 percent milk: 0.82 to 8.98 mcg
- Yogurt: 4.32 mcg
- Cheese pizza (This receives an executive pardon from Dr. Ray, by the way.); 5.46 to 7.10 mcg

The average of these values shows almost double the amount of lead in dairy compared with the many calcium supplements on the market. In addition, the protein in milk acts as a carrier molecule for the lead. This results in an increase in lead absorption (*Food, Cosmetics, and Toxicology.* 13:555–63). Suddenly, the lead content of calcium supplements becomes trivial, especially if the supplement is replacing dairy intake.

Calcium's Limitations

It is important to know that calcium is only one piece of the osteoporotic puzzle. There are at least 12 minerals that are essential in the proper formation of healthy bones. Conventional medicine would have you believe that the story ends with calcium. They are mistaken. There is so much more to the picture.

A study published in 1979 in the *American Journal of Clinical Nutrition* looked at two closely related groups of people in Yugoslavia. One group from the Podravia district spent a lot of time indoors and drank lots of dairy products, which provided an average daily intake of approximately 900 mg of calcium. The people from the Istra district did more farming and thus spent more time in the sun, ate more vegetables, and worked hard in the fields. Their intake of calcium was a paltry 400 mg per day.

When scientists looked at the risk of fracture over a 6-year period, they were surprised to find that the people from the Istra district suffered less than half of the incidence of hip fracture (104 versus

225), despite consuming just 400 mg of calcium daily. This example simply illustrates the fact that calcium is only one small piece of the puzzle; it even appears to take a back seat to other, more important factors, which we will discuss in detail in the coming sections (*AJCN*.1979:540–549).

Supplements Reduce Deaths After Hip Fracture

After someone fractures a hip, the outlook is quite grim, with 2 out of 10 patients dying within one year. A small study performed in 2009 found that the patients who supplemented with calcium and vitamin D after the fracture fared much better than those who failed to supplement. In fact, male participants who consistently took their calcium and vitamin D enjoyed a 43 percent reduction in death rates; female subjects enjoyed a 36 percent reduction in the death rate. Women who took their supplements along with anti-osteoporosis medications enjoyed a similar reduction as the men who took supplements alone (43 percent). This amounts to just a 7 percent decrease compared with the women who took supplements alone.

In the section to follow, we will discuss other supplements that can be of great use in your fight against osteoporosis. We will start with one of the most important: vitamin D.

Are Calcium Supplements Causing Heart Attacks?

In case you have not heard, the press has been reporting that calcium supplements are causing your arteries to become calcified.

So, I will bet you are wondering if it is true …

Well, let us look at the most recent study that had practically every newsroom and paper reporting that calcium supplements increase your risk of heart attack by 86 percent. First, you must know that the study was performed in Germany, the world's central command in the war against natural medicine. It is the model for all the anti-nutrition legislature that big pharma has been trying to get passed here in the United States. So far, they have been unsuccessful, but I will be keeping a close eye on them. Just know that the country where the study was performed (Germany) is no friend of nutritional medicine, which speaks to bias.

In this study, the researchers evaluated data from 23,980 participants over an 11-year period. In this group of nearly 24,000 people, 851 were using calcium supplements or calcium-containing supplements. To show you just how poorly designed this study was, the calcium takers were more likely to be smokers and to have high cholesterol. This means that the people in the study who were taking calcium were already at higher risk of heart disease—which likely accounts for any negative findings in the study.

In addition, because of the small number of people taking calcium supplements, the researchers had to massage the data in order to come up with that 86 percent number.

As Mark Twain said, "If you torture statistics long enough, you can get them to say whatever you want them to say."

And torture them they did …

Do you remember the clinical term for this type of research? If you guessed "hogwash," then you get the prize. So, now that we have established that this study is junk-science (the actual term), I do have concerns about how many doctors prescribe calcium supplements, since it violates what nature wants …

First, calcium alone will not save your bones. Every single day I speak to people who have been told by their doctors to take 1,500 mg to 2,000 mg of calcium per day. That is just plain ridiculous.

I like to say that you cannot build a house with wood alone, that you need many other building blocks, such as plaster, nails, wiring, glass, plastic, etc. Likewise, bones are comprised of many different components. Sure, calcium is the most abundant mineral, but just because wood makes up the majority of a house does not mean the nails are less important.

Bones need calcium, magnesium, boron, zinc, manganese, silica, and more. So, I recommend supplementing with a bone mineral formula rather than with calcium alone.

In addition, I have concerns that huge doses of calcium may suppress the activation of vitamin D, which may have negative health consequences. Vitamin D acts more like a hormone in the body than a vitamin. It has many effects within the body, beyond simply increasing the absorption of minerals. Interfering with the activation of vitamin D could negatively affect the cardiovascular system, the brain, and the immune system.

Finally, you can have too much of anything, including water. Do not drown yourself in any single mineral, including calcium. Stick to the guidelines in the program: 400 to 800 mg is likely safe and effective. Most people should not supplement with more than 1,000 mg of calcium daily.

Chapter Summary

Dairy is not the savior to the bones that the dairy industry would have you believe. The countries with the highest dairy intake also suffer the highest incidence of osteoporosis. Likewise, calcium alone will not save your bones. You need a blend of mineral building blocks that all work together to keep the bones healthy. Avoid calcium carbonate as it neutralizes the stomach acid and is the least absorbed calcium supplement; choose MCHA, amino acid chelated calcium, citrate, or citrate-malate as these forms absorb best. Avoid mega doses of calcium, stick to a maximum of 500 to 800 mg per day and balance it with equal amounts of magnesium if you suffer from calcium-induced constipation.

10

A Vitamin D-Ficient Society

The Science of Vitamin D

Here is the bottom line: low vitamin D equates to poor calcium absorption and higher parathyroid hormone levels. You have three ways of getting vitamin D into your system: Your body's primary source is from the conversion of cholesterol into vitamin D. This process takes place when sunlight strikes the skin and triggers the conversion reaction. The second way is through the intake of foods naturally containing or fortified with vitamin D, such as fish, oils, eggs, liver, and milk (*New England Journal Medicine.*

326:1213,1992). The final source of vitamin D is through supplementation. If vitamin D is as abundant as sunlight, why are we D-ficient? There are numerous reasons:

- Adam and Eve ate the apple. This was the first day we started wearing clothes that block the sun from striking our natural solar panel: the skin.
- We live in a sunphobic society: sunscreen, tinted windows, hats, and even sunscreen-laced clothing. With the advances in science, it seems we have become walking, breathing "shade."
- We have a cholesterol-lowering obsession. Less cholesterol equates to fewer building blocks for vitamin D. If you want a surefire way to lower cholesterol, get regular exposure to the sun.
- There are seasonal changes. In the winter, sun exposure plummets, exacerbating the deficiency further (*J Am Geriatr Soc,* 45(5): 598–603 1997 May).

- Vitamin D can be sequestered by fat cells. The heavier we get, the less vitamin D we have available to the body.

Vitamin D deficiency causes two main problems with bone health: As vitamin D levels decrease, so does the absorption of calcium from supplements and food. Second, parathyroid levels increase, leading to leaching of calcium from the bone. These are likely two important ways by which vitamin D deficiency impacts bone health. However, it should be noted that more and more research is constantly being published about vitamin D, and I believe we will see other important roles of vitamin D in bone, cardiovascular, and metabolic health.

Some recent discoveries show that vitamin D appears to help osteoblasts absorb calcium, thus giving them ammunition to build bones. In addition, vitamin D appears to block a compound called c-fos that stimulates the production and activation of new osteoclasts (bone-breaking cells) (*J Clin Invest*, February 2006).

Scientists in Italy recently discovered one additional mechanism of vitamin D: They cultured osteoblasts (bone-building cells) from healthy bones and osteoporotic bones of elderly subjects and then exposed the bone-building cells to identical levels of vitamin D in a laboratory. The scientists discovered that vitamin D does not appear to stimulate much activity in the bones of elderly osteoporotic patients compared with those having healthy bones. This may mean that "average" levels of vitamin D may be insufficient in elderly subjects with osteoporosis. In fact, they may require higher levels of vitamin D than younger subjects with healthier bone cells (*Rheumatology International,* 2009;29(6):667–672). I call this issue "vitamin D resistance," which may explain why some people are more prone to osteoporosis.

Vitamin D Controversy – Isn't Vitamin D Toxic?

In 1948 there were case reports of vitamin D toxicity. Even though these cases occurred because of vitamin D consumption between 150,000 to 600,000 IU of vitamin D (the government suggests 600 IU daily), the damage was done. To date, practitioners have been afraid to go above 1,000 IU of vitamin D daily. A detailed report published in 1999 showed that vitamin D is safe at doses up to 10,000 IU daily and most effective at a dose of at least 4,000 IU every day. However, I should point out that each person is unique in how much vitamin D they need.

Total body exposure to the midday sunlight would cause you to produce 10,000 IU of vitamin D. Toxicity may occur at doses greater than 40,000 IU daily (*AJCN*, Vol. 69, No. 5, 842–56, May 1999). William Campbell Douglas, MD, noted that researchers at the University of Chicago have found vitamin D to be among the safest vitamins available. Dr. Douglas suggests osteoporotic patients should take a daily dose of 5,000 IU of vitamin D (*What They're Not Telling You About Osteoporosis.* Second Opinion

Publishing, 1997). The reason vitamin D is so safe is because the human body appears to have mechanisms within its skin to prevent excess production of vitamin D. When vitamin D reaches a certain concentration in the body, sun exposure then becomes a mechanism for breaking down excessive vitamin D rather than a catalyst for vitamin D production.

Action to Take:

Studies have shown that the body is capable of producing 10,000 IU of vitamin D, provided you get full-body exposure to unblocked summer sun (such as while wearing a Speedo or string bikini). Unfortunately, there are a number of factors that can decrease your body's ability to produce vitamin D, including:

- Being dark-skinned
- Being obese
- Being vegetarian
- Being too self-conscious to wear a Speedo or string bikini
- Using sunscreen

- Taking cholesterol-blocking medications

Also, it is important to note that the body will activate vitamin D in the liver and kidney. Vitamin D produced by sun exposure or taken in through nutritional supplement is carried to the liver and converted into 25-OH-vitamin D, which is two to five times more active in the body than the original vitamin D building block. The 25-OH-vitamin D is then carried to the kidneys, where it is further activated into the most potent form called 1,25-OH-vitamin D. If either or both of these organs are not functioning properly, then you will see a decrease in the effectiveness of vitamin D.

The evidence is clear that vitamin D is safe at doses up to 10,000 IU daily in the general population. However, research has shown that doses greater than 4,000 IU are unnecessary in the average person, unless your blood tests show otherwise. In a study, subjects who received 4,000 IU of vitamin D_3 for 14 days showed blood levels of the vitamin increased dramatically, while remaining well within the safe ranges. This study compared the effects of vitamin D_3 (natural) to vitamin D_2 (synthetic). Vitamin D_2 is a less expensive form that, in my opinion, is unsuitable for human consumption. Research in the past has used this inferior form of vitamin D and shown negative results with bone density —I am not surprised. In this study, vitamin D_3 raised blood levels of the vitamin 1.7 times higher than an equivalent dose of vitamin D_2. Not to mention the fact that the body does not know what to do with this synthetic form (*AJCN.* 68:854–858. 1998).

Vitamins D_2 and D_3 are not created equal in the body; in fact, they share different pathways of metabolism. In the human body, there are proteins that act as the taxi, carrying the precious vitamin D compounds to the various tissues of the body. Research has determined that the protein carriers of vitamin D prefer natural vitamin D_3 to the metabolites of synthetic vitamin D_2. This explains why such high doses of the synthetic are required and why even at these high doses most people still do not respond.

Vitamin D_3 is still only pennies a day. A total of 800 IU daily of vitamin D has shown significant reductions in risk of non-vertebral fractures (30 percent decrease) and the incidence of hip fractures (41 percent decrease); 400 IU daily showed no protection from fractures when administered to elderly patients (*BMJ,* November 28, 1998; 317: 1466-1467; *Nutr Review.*51 (1993):183–85).

Thus, to improve the health of your skeleton, I suggest doses of 2,000 to 4,000 IU of vitamin D daily for most people. We find that the combined amounts of vitamin D from a high-quality bone mineral formula, a high-quality multivitamin, and moderate exposure to the sun may meet this vitamin D requirement. Many times, however, extra D supplementation may be required. Our recommendation is to get started on a program like this now to avoid having osteoporosis problems later.

To aggressively improve and maintain optimal bone density, doses of up to

4,000 IU of vitamin D can be used safely. Less vitamin D is produced in dark-skinned individuals, and thus they may need to dose at higher levels than light-skinned individuals. Younger people produce more vitamin D than older folks and thus can get away with a lower dose (1,000 mg to 2,000 IU) vitamin D. We find that people with a current osteoporosis issue may need to add extra vitamin D to the multivitamin and bone mineral formula that they already take. And, of course, a little extra exposure to the sun (early morning or late afternoon are the safest times) would serve to fill in any shortfall from the supplementation.

There is still a lot of controversy regarding whether vitamin D levels can be met through sun exposure alone. In an interesting study, researchers from the University of Wisconsin Osteoporosis Clinical Research Program found that vitamin D levels remained inadequate even in people who receive significant amounts of sun. In this study of people living in Hawaii, the average subject spent 22.4 hours in the sun without sunscreen and a total of 28.9 hours with and without sunscreen during the course of the study. This translates into 11.1 hours per week of total body sun exposure. Despite this abundant level of sun exposure, over half of the subjects had serum levels of vitamin D below 30 ng/ml, which indicates a deficiency. This study demonstrates that the recommended 15 minutes per day of sun exposure is not sufficient to meet the demands of the bones (*J Clin Endocrinol Metab.* 2007;92:2130–2135).

If You Are Overweight, Read This

If you carry extra weight, you will likely require extra vitamin D due to the fact that vitamin D in your bloodstream will be commandeered by fat cells. This fat-sequestering phenomenon may explain why there is such variance in blood levels of vitamin D between people who take supplements even though the vitamin D dose may be the same (*J Clin Endocrinol Metab.* 88:157–161,2003).

If you are overweight, I highly recommend getting blood tests to assess your vitamin D status. It is extremely difficult to estimate the appropriate dose in people who carry extra fat tissue. In the absence of such a test, I would recommend taking 10,000 IU of vitamin D_3 per day for two weeks, followed by a daily dose of 5,000 IU daily thereafter. More may be needed if blood tests continue to show inadequate vitamin D levels.

How to increase Vitamin D without taking Vitamin D or exposing yourself to sunlight

The complexity of the body never ceases to amaze me. In a study published in 2008, researchers examined the effect of antioxidants and aerobic exercise on bone metabolism. Thirteen seniors were given 500 mg of vitamin C and 100 mg of vitamin E and then placed on a supervised aerobic exercise program. After eight weeks, it was discovered that vitamin D levels increased by 42.8 percent, PTH decreased by 17.5 percent, and one marker of bone breakdown (alkaline phosphatase) decreased by 14.6 percent. The researchers concluded that the antioxidants, along with aerobic exercise, resulted in improved metabolism of vitamin D and PTH. Ultimately, this is expected to improve bone quality and density (*J Sports Science.* 26:251–258, 2008).

The body is a web of complexity. Plucking even just one string on that web results in a reverberation throughout the entire web. We must be careful not to overconcentrate our efforts by focusing on one nutrient, food, or lifestyle change. This study simply confirms this philosophy.

Vitamin D Works Synergistically with Vitamin K

Vitamins D and K work together to improve bone mass. When vitamin D is added to vitamin K supplementation, then bone-building cells are activated to a greater degree (*J Clin Endocrinol Metab.*

1999 Aug; 84(8):2700–2704). We will discuss vitamin K later in the book.

Despite the past controversy, vitamin D appears to be a very safe supplement when taken in doses up to 5,000 IU daily. Some people will require more, and some will need less. Regardless, it is clear that vitamin D is a critical component of your bone-resilience plan. If you have blood testing performed to evaluate vitamin D, we consider anything below 30 ng/ml to put you in the red zone, 31 to 49 ng/ml in the yellow zone, and 50 to 70 ng/ml in the green/optimal zone. If your blood tests shows levels above 70 ng/ml, we recommend cutting the dose back until you reach a level of 50 to 70 ng/ml. As always, seek the help of a qualified healthcare provider.

Chapter Summary:

Vitamin D is considered one of the safest and most important vitamins for building healthy bones. Although doctors will commonly prescribe vitamin D_2, research suggests that vitamin D_3 is safer and more effective. Dosing requirements can vary depending on the person's sun exposure, body weight, age, and race thus blood tests for vitamin D may be necessary to determine the appropriate dose. Vitamin D works synergistically with vitamin K.

11

The Supporting Actors - Minerals That Matter

Magnesium – Add a Little Bounce to the Bones

Magnesium is believed to be as important to bone health as calcium. Researchers believe that up to 80 percent of the American population has some degree of magnesium deficiency (*JAMA*. 263: 3063, 1990). Preliminary studies found that women who are osteoporotic have lower bone magnesium levels and show other signs of magnesium deficiency compared with nonosteoporotic populations (*Isr J Med Sci.* 1981;17:1123–1125).

Many osteoporotic patients can have a deficiency of the most active form of vitamin D called 1,25-(OH)-Vitamin D, which is 10 times more active than vitamin D produced by the sun or taken in via supplement. Magnesium plays an important role in converting inactive vitamin D from the sun or supplement into the activated form that results in stronger bones.

In a small study, magnesium supplements were given to 19 postmenopausal women with low bone density who were on estrogen replacement therapy. After one year of magnesium supplementation, 12 of the study subjects no longer had low bone density (*J Reprod Med.* 35:503, 1990). Magnesium supplementation has been associated with a 1.0 to 8.0 percent increase in bone density (*Magnesium Research.* 6: 155, 1993). In young, healthy males, magnesium supplementation resulted in decreases in markers of bone loss and PTH levels. No changes in calcium levels were noted in the blood. This shows that even in young, healthy males there is a benefit from magnesium supplementation (*J Clin Endocrinol Metab,* Aug 1998, 83(8) 2742–8).

Another study evaluated the importance of magnesium in helping young girls develop healthy bones. Fifty girls ages 8 to 14 with a history of low magnesium intake were split into two groups: One group received 300 mg of magnesium daily; the other group received a placebo. After one year, the girls who received the magnesium had a 3 percent greater bone density in the hips. The authors reported that "[t]his study provides data supporting the idea that magnesium supplementation has positive effects on accrual of bone mass in adolescents with suboptimal magnesium intake" (*J Clin Endocrinol Metab.* 2006 Dec;91(12):4866–72).

Everybody claims to have the "magical ratio" of calcium to magnesium —anywhere from 4:1 to 1:1. Who is right?

Whenever we come across a question like this we look toward nature for the answer. The truth is, calcium and magnesium come in a variety of ratios in different foods. Our diet, however, is more abundant in calcium and deficient in magnesium due to fortification. In my opinion, bone health would suffer if we consume more than a 2:1 ratio of calcium to magnesium. So get enough magnesium to get at least a 2:1 ratio of calcium to magnesium as a minimum. Given the relative abundance of calcium in our "fortified" diet, the likelihood is that magnesium is a more likely deficiency. So, I generally recommend that you aim to get a ratio closer to 1:1. This means that in supplement form, you may want to get 100 mg of magnesium for each 100 mg of calcium.

The fact is that the abundance of calcium in the diet will likely result in a ratio of 2:1 when dietary calcium is taken into account. Care should be taken in calculating the net effect of all the calcium and magnesium coming from a multivitamin and bone mineral formula with respect to this ratio. Extra magnesium (we suggest magnesium citrate, glycinate, aspartate, or orotate) can be taken to adjust the amounts.

Calcium and magnesium can be taken together or separately. Although there is evidence that calcium may compete for absorption with magnesium, copper, zinc, and other minerals, I do not believe that it is significant enough to require separation. In my experience, people who take the minerals separately have a much harder time being consistent.

Phosphorus

Phosphorus is the second most abundant mineral in the body, second only to calcium. Eighty to 90 percent of the phosphorus is found in the bones. Much like calcium, absorption, storage, and extraction of phosphorous are dependent on vitamin D and PTH. The suggested intake of phosphorus is believed to be a 1:1 ratio with calcium; however, phosphorus is more abundant in a standard human diet than calcium. Thus, a 2:1 ratio of calcium to phosphorus is more logical. This ratio is the same found in bones and is the natural ratio found in bone meal, such as MCHA. Dietary sources of phosphorus include meat and soda (Lieberman, S. *The Real Vitamin & Mineral Book* 2nd Edition. Avery. 1997).

Phosphorous is a double-edged sword. Researchers have found that having a 3:1 ratio of phosphorous to calcium (1,500 mg of phosphorous to 500 mg of calcium) can significantly increase PTH and thus promote osteoporosis. Carbonated drinks are one of the most harmful sources of phosphorous in our diet.

For the most part, I would not make an effort to supplement with phosphorous. My research suggests that most of us have enough in the diet to meet the body's needs. It is fine if you get a bit more from your bone supplements, but there is no need to take it as a separate supplement.

Strontium As A Bone-Building Supplement

Strontium is a trace mineral found naturally in the human body in small quantities. In recent years, strontium has been studied as a tool for increasing bone density. Results have been quite impressive as strontium has resulted in an increase in bone density, increase in bone formation, and decrease in fracture risk. The majority of the research has been performed on a form of strontium called strontium ranelate. It is important to note that the "ranelate" portion has no activity in the bones; it is the strontium that seems to impact them. It appears that researchers chose this form of strontium because it can be patented and then sold as a medication. Other forms of strontium should provide similar benefits. Forms that can be found in health-food stores include strontium citrate and strontium carbonate.

Strontium, like many health-related products, has two sides to the coin. Below, I will provide some of the advantages and disadvantages of this trace mineral. As for the advantages, I have already touched on them in the previous paragraph. First, strontium is a natural product found in food and water. Second, strontium appears to have a fairly high level of short-term safety, with studies showing doses up to 1,750 mg per day to be free of side effects. Third, strontium has been shown to increase the activity of bone-building cells rather than simply interfering with the bone-breaking cells. Finally, strontium has been found to decrease the risk of bone fracture.

Now, let us talk about some of the potential disadvantages. First, strontium is a trace mineral that appears to occur in the diet in amounts that rarely exceed 3 mg daily. However, supplementation will usually call for between 170 to 680 mg of strontium daily. This could throw off the balance of other minerals in the body. Second, strontium seems to compete for absorption with minerals, such as calcium and magnesium. Third, strontium appears to affect bones only at a surface level, and the benefits seem to reverse themselves quickly after supplementation is ceased. Fourth, there appears to be controversy as to the optimal dosage of strontium, with one study showing better results with fracture risk if 170 mg is used instead of 680 mg. Finally, strontium supplementation may interfere with the proper interpretation of DXA scans, making the bones appear denser than they actually are.

Bottom Line:

In a previous section of this book, we evaluated the importance of magnesium on bone health. Some researchers believe that strontium is acting as a surrogate for magnesium when magnesium is deficient. If this is true, then it is more important that we correct magnesium deficiency than to provide the body with high, unnatural doses of strontium. Although strontium appears to provide benefits to bones in the short term, we just do not know if the net long-term result after years of supplementation is positive or negative. Thus, it is my recommendation that strontium is used as a tool only for people who have significant/severe osteoporosis that places them at a high risk of fracture. For everybody else, including those with osteopenia and mild to /early-stage osteoporosis, I would recommend avoiding this supplement in high doses until more data becomes available. Strontium can be kept in the toolbox but should be reserved for those who are in grave danger or who have tried everything else without result. I feel that taking strontium in amounts found in a healthy diet—3 to 6 mg per day—is fine and likely healthy. For now, however, hold off on the high, pharmaceutical doses until more data is available.

"Tracing" the Path to Healthy bones

In addition to macrominerals (minerals required in high levels), our bones rely on trace minerals found in the human body in minute quantities, including boron, silica, manganese, selenium, zinc, strontium, and copper. In a 2-year, double-blind study, postmenopausal women were given either a placebo, calcium citrate alone, trace minerals alone, or calcium and trace minerals together. The only significant change occurred in the group given the calcium and trace minerals together. In the placebo group, there was a bone density decline of 3 percent; in the calcium alone group, there was a decrease of 1.25 percent; a 1.89 percent decline in the trace mineral group; and in the group given both calcium and trace minerals, a 1.48 percent increase in bone density was found. The trace minerals given were zinc (15 mg), manganese (5 mg), and copper (2.5 mg) (*J Nutr.* Jul 1994; 124(7):1060–4).

In a study of postmenopausal women, 3 mg of boron supplementation daily resulted in a lesser excretion of magnesium and calcium. The researchers also noted an increase in estrogen and testosterone levels in women taking boron. Estrogen is believed to help decrease bone loss, while testosterone is believed to help stimulate bone formation. In women for whom elevated estrogen levels are not desired, increasing magnesium levels will minimize the elevation of estrogen production. This would be especially beneficial for women who have had breast cancer (*FASEB J.* Nov 1987; 1(5): 394–7).

Research at Emory University Department of Medicine suggests that zinc may be especially important in the repair and development of a healthy skeleton. Scientists found that increased zinc within the bone structure was correlated with decreased bone aging and increased bone resiliency. They made note that zinc appears to stimulate the bone-building cells, which results in enhanced mineralization of the bone (*Mol Cell Biochem.* Dec 2009).

Science has a tendency to focus its attention on the compounds found to be most abundant in nature; the belief being, if the diet contains higher quantities then it must be more important. We made this crude mistake when we assumed that alpha-tocopherol was the only vitamin E that was important to health because it was the most abundant. The fact that other forms of vitamin E were found in smaller quantities caused scientists to ignore them. It turns out that this was a grave mistake. These other, less abundant, forms of vitamin E are now believed to be of equal or greater importance. Trace minerals are no different, with their tiny quantities making them easy to overlook. Although large-scale studies have not been completed, I feel that it would be a mistake to ignore these vital microminerals provided they are consumed in amounts that would naturally be found in a healthy diet.

The Healthiest Table Salt on Earth

Sodium intake in our society is way out of hand. Even worse, our lack of potassium intake has resulted in a severe imbalance in the sodium and potassium levels of our bodies. Harvard researchers have discovered that the sodium/potassium ratio, assessed by urinalysis, could be a good predictor of cardiovascular disease risk. The higher the sodium intake and the lower the potassium intake, the higher the risk of cardiovascular disease.

Recent research has found that simply replacing table salt with a potassium-rich table salt could significantly decrease the risk of heart disease. A nationwide study performed in Finland replaced sodium-rich salt with a special salt blend that instead contained: potassium, magnesium, and l-lysine. This special blend appears to have resulted in as much as a 65 percent drop in cardiovascular death risk throughout the country. That is nothing short of astounding.

So, what does this have to do with bones?

Although bones and osteoporosis risk were not part of this Finnish study; the special salt formula used contains two minerals that are critical for healthy bones. We have discussed magnesium, and potassium will be discussed later. Using this special salt is a wonderful way to start balancing the sodium/potassium ratio while providing the body with much-needed magnesium. By using this salt in place of sodium-rich salt, you may protect your bones *and* your heart.

The salt formula is now available in the United States under the name

GoodSalt. It is fairly inexpensive and very tasty.

Chapter Summary:

A complete bone-building program should include supporting minerals such as magnesium, phosphorous, and other trace minerals. Strontium is commonly promoted for helping to reverse osteoporosis, however, research has questioned the safety and efficacy of longterm, high-dose strontium supplementation. For that reason I recommend avoiding high doses of strontium (limit supplementation to 6 mg or less) until more research is published proving strontium's safety in high doses for extended periods of time.

12

Inflammation & Medications - Enemies of the Skeleton

Inflammation Contributes to Osteoporosis

In recent years, more and more information has come to light around how inflammation impacts bone loss. Researchers at Purdue University discovered that certain inflammatory compounds in the body called prostaglandins and leukotrienes could stimulate the bone-removing cells (osteoclasts) to destroy otherwise healthy bone. Research has found that the best way to decrease inflammation in the body is by eating foods that decrease inflammation, by lessening the stress in your life, and by using certain supplements, such as essential fatty acids.

Essential Fats – We Are Not Just Skin and Bones

Essential fatty acids (EFAs) help protect the heart, decrease inflammation in the body, build healthy joints, enhance skin quality, improve immune function, and maintain a healthy mood. Recent evidence has confirmed another well-known benefit of EFAs: building and maintaining healthy bones. Fish oil, for example, has been shown to decrease urinary calcium excretion. Animal studies have demonstrated that EFA deficiency leads to severe osteoporosis, renal calcification (kidney stones), and arteriosclerosis (hardening of the arteries). In another animal study, GLA (primrose and borage oil) and EPA (fish oil) was given to animals who then showed a 41 percent increase in intestinal absorption of calcium compared with no increase in the placebo group. In elderly women given GLA and EPA, there was a decrease in two markers of bone breakdown: osteocalcin and deoxypyridinoline. After 18 months, there was an increase in thigh bone density (3.1 percent increase) and spinal (lumbar) bone density (4.7 percent increase). The EFAs have also demonstrated a significant ability to decrease inflammatory chemicals in the blood that lead to increased bone breakdown and decreased bone building (*Nutrition.* 2000;16:386–390).

In an interesting study, researchers put subjects on three different diets containing various amounts of fats:

- Standard American Diet, containing 34 percent total fat, 13 percent saturated fat, 13 percent monounsaturated fat, and 9 percent polyunsaturated fat (7.7 percent omega-6 and 0.8 percent omega-3 as alpha-linolenic acid)

- Inflammatory Fat Diet high in linoleic acid, containing 37 percent total fat, 9 percent saturated fat, 12 percent monounsaturated fat, and 16 percent polyunsaturated fat (12.6 percent omega-6 and 3.6 percent omega-3 fatty acids from alpha-lipoic acid)
- Anti-inflammatory Diet, containing 38 percent total fat, 8 percent saturated fat, 12 percent monounsaturated fat, and 17 percent polyunsaturated fat (10.5 percent omega-6 and 6.5 percent omega-3)

The group was placed on each diet for six weeks and tested for N-telopeptides to determine how much bone was being broken down. The main sources of omega-3 fatty acids were flaxseed oil and walnuts. The group that was placed on the high omega-3 fatty acid diet showed significantly lower N-telopeptides compared with the other two groups, with the highest bone breakdown being in the standard American diet group. The lower the N-telopeptide level, the healthier the bone is (less bone loss and more bone formation) (*Nutr J,* 2007;6(1):2).

Research at Purdue University has also discovered that high doses of fish oil could help to decrease levels of certain inflammatory pro-hormones called PGE2. This finding is just one more confirmation that diet and supplementation with omega-3 fats could protect bones.

Antioxidants... As Effective as Resistance Exercise?

A Canadian study evaluated the impact of a very basic antioxidant blend containing 1,000 mg of vitamin C along with 600 mg of vitamin E on bone loss. The antioxidants were compared within a group given a placebo, a group that was placed on a resistance exercise program, and a group given a combination of antioxidants and resistance exercise. After six months, the placebo group saw a decrease in bone density of the spine, while the subjects placed on the resistance exercise and antioxidants enjoyed a stable bone density with no appreciable loss. This pilot study suggests that antioxidants may play an important role in the prevention of osteoporosis. Does this mean that you can pop an antioxidant pill instead of hitting the gym? Sorry, not going to find permission in this book. We will get into exercise later, but I think you will see the value of resistance exercise and hope that you will make it a permanent part of your bone-building program (*Osteoporos Int,* 2008 Nov 20).

Back to Magnesium…

In a University of California, Los Angeles, study published in the journal *Diabetes Care,* researchers discovered that magnesium is a powerful anti-inflammatory nutrient. In this study on 3,713 postmenopausal women, each 100 mg increase in magnesium resulted in cumulative decreases in various measures of inflammation, such as CRP, TNFa, and Interleukin 6. This is just one more example of how magnesium can benefit the bones as well as the rest of the body (*Diabetes Care.* 2009 November).

We Have a Bone to Pick with the Drugs

There are numerous drugs that can cause further depletion of vital nutrients from the bones:

Prednisone & Steroids

It is no secret among healthcare practitioners that continued use of even low-dose steroids, such as prednisone (Deltasone®), can lead to a deterioration of bone. That is the reason prednisone is supposed to be used as a last line agent and only for short periods of time. Unfortunately, this drug has been used more often than it should with many people; in some cases it is the only drug that can provide relief from a condition from which they suffer (such as certain autoimmune conditions). For these people, we have good news:

Supplementing with calcium and vitamin D can stop bone loss and even lead to bone growth in people who must use this powerful anti-inflammatory. A 2-year, double-blind study involving 96 rheumatoid arthritis patients on chronic low-dose prednisone therapy was performed. One group received calcium carbonate (1,000mg per day) and vitamin D (500 IU), while the other group received a placebo. The group receiving the placebo showed continued loss of bone mass over the study period (2 percent loss in the lumbar spine and 0.9 percent per year in the thigh bone). The group receiving the calcium and vitamin D_3 gained 0.72 percent of bone mass per year in the lumbar spine and 0.85 percent in the thigh bone (*Ann Intern Med,* 125(12): 961–8. 1996). These results were achieved using an inferior form of calcium and an inferior dose of vitamin D_3. What results would we have seen if we had given higher-dose vitamin D_3, a full bone-mineral formula, and a bone - building exercise plan? Imagine what we could have achieved with a complete bone-resiliency program.

Diuretics

Diuretics—what most people call "water pills"—are used to take fluid out of the body, thus decreasing blood pressure. Unfortunately, these drugs can also cause a depletion of such minerals as potassium, magnesium, and calcium. The biggest culprit is a drug called furosemide (Lasix®). This is a powerful diuretic that can cause depletion of calcium and, more importantly, be associated with a higher risk of osteoporosis and fracture (*Nord Med.* 113(2): 53–9 1998 Feb). The thiazide diuretics, such as hydrochlorothiazide (HCTZ), do not cause this depletion of calcium; as a matter of fact, they may even prevent osteoporosis by preventing calcium loss (*Osteoporos Int.* 7(1):79–84 1997). Although thiazine diuretics do not deplete calcium, they can deplete potassium over time; your doctor should monitor potassium levels and treat deficiency accordingly. A worrisome downside of all diuretics is that they can increase nighttime urination, resulting in groggy trips to the bathroom in the dark, which places people at a higher risk of falls.

Cimetidine (Tagamet)

This medication is used to decrease the amount of acid being produced by the stomach. As mentioned earlier, the decrease in stomach acid production can lead to a decrease in calcium absorption. In addition, this medication has been shown to decrease your body's ability to utilize vitamin D (*J Lab Clin Med.* 1984, 104(4):546–52).

Acid Reflux Drugs (Aciphex®, Nexium®, Prevacid®, Prilosec)

In a University of Pennsylvania study published in the *Journal of the American Medical Association,* people over age 50 who took acid reflux drugs called proton pump inhibitors (or PPIs, as discussed previously) saw a 44 percent increased risk of breaking a hip. People who took these medications long term saw a 245 percent increased risk of hip fracture. The higher the dose, the higher the risk of bone fractures. It is hypothesized that these medications inhibit calcium absorption by inhibiting stomach acid production.

Antidepressant Medications (Zoloft®, Prozac®, etc.)

Bone fracture has been a long-known but rarely publicized side effect of medications used to treat depression. In fact, a 2007 study published in the *Archives of Internal Medicine* found that these medications actually double the risk of bone fracture. Even though dizziness and low blood pressure are common side effects of this class of medication and can result in falls, the risk of fracture was found to be independent of these effects. In other words, antidepressants may actually make the bones weaker while increasing the risk of falls. This is a very disturbing side effect and one that should spur further research. If you are currently taking medications for depression, please be sure that these medications are a necessary tool. Always discuss the risks and benefits with your doctor.

It should also be noted that research has linked depression itself with low bone mineral density. As a matter of fact, current or past depression could result in a 6 percent loss of bone density in the spine and a whopping 14 percent decrease in density of the hips.

Chapter Summary:

Many drugs can interfere with the formation of strong, resilient bone. These drugs act as a "resistance factor" interferes with your body's ability to manufacture a healthy bone matrix. Always ask your doctor or pharmacist if prescribed medications may negatively impact your bones and seek alternatives when feasible.

13

Exercising Your Right to Strong Bones

Introduction to Exercise for Building Bones

If I were to throw a pile of wood, nails, and tools in front of you and say, "Go!" the first thing out of your mouth would be "Go do what?" Is this not what we do to our bodies? We throw a thousand wonderful building blocks at our body and give it no stimulus to build. The old physics adage holds true with our body: an object at rest tends to stay at rest. Our body resists energy expenditure unless there is some call for it. If we do not stress the bones in a way that makes them want to grow stronger, then there is no reason for the body to build strong bones. It would simply be a waste of energy. We call that the Law of Need: your bones are as strong as they need to be, given the stresses they are exposed to on a regular basis. Whenever the bones are put through enough stress (load-bearing exercise), calcium phosphate crystals in the bone cause a small electric charge, called a "piezoelectric effect," which appears to stimulate the bone-building cells to lay down bone matrix in the areas of stress. Without regular mechanical stress to the body, the bone-removing cells receive messages to get rid of the unnecessary bone and start chomping away at the bone—both the brittle and the good, healthy bone. By living a sedentary life, a slow and steady bone erosion occurs because the normal bone-removing process continues without stimulating the bone-building cells to counter the loss.

Studies have been done to evaluate the impact of activity and exercise on bone mass. Here are a few facts that researchers have discovered:

1. Men who exercise vigorously have 14 percent higher trabecular bone mass (inner bone) than those who do not exercise.
2. Among athletes, the more vigorous the activity, the higher the bone density, especially in athletes that do a lot of jumping and sprinting.
3. Among women who are not athletic, those who were more active in everyday life enjoyed higher bone density than those who were not as active.
4. People who have more active work have higher bone density than those with sedentary jobs.
5. Single-limb-dominant athletes, such as tennis players, have a tendency to have higher density in the arm that is involved in the activity.

Researchers at the Mayo Clinic put one group of osteoporotic women on a workout routine comprised of simple back exercises and compared them with a control group. After several years of follow-up, just 16 percent of the women in the workout group suffered new spinal fractures compared with 67 percent in the control (no exercise) group (*Arch Phys Med Rehab.* 65 (1984): 593–596).

Research at the University of Connecticut Health Center suggests that an exercise program can increase bone density by 5 to 10 percent. According to this research, the worse your bone density, the bigger the gains in bone mass. This just goes to show you that the body wants strong bones—, that is, when it is given the appropriate stimulus (*Compr-Thor,* Sept:15 (1989):30–37).

Inactivity – The Scourge of Your Bones

Let us look at the opposite spectrum, known in medicine as "Couch and Bonbon Syndrome." We know that astronauts can spend weeks in space and return with significantly lower bone density, losing 1 to 3 percent of their bone mass each month in space. We know that people on bed rest can end up with severe osteoporosis. In fact, people who are on bed rest can lose up to 1 percent of the bone density in their spines each week (*Clin Science*. 64 (1983):537–540).

One way that I can tell if someone has good bone strength is to assess his or her physical strength. Research has shown that bone mass correlates well with muscle strength; the stronger the muscles, the stronger the bones. As we age, muscle mass can erode, and the bones follow suit.

The simple message here is, move it or lose it. Weakness is a global problem in the body; it is never localized in the muscles.

What Kind of Exercise Will Build Bone?

Weight-bearing exercise and strength-training exercise are the answer. Any exercise that puts weight or stress on the bones has the potential to improve the upkeep of the skeleton. Weight-bearing exercise means any activity that involves lugging around your own weight, which can be as simple as walking. In a study of postmenopausal women, the sedentary group lost on average 7 percent of their bone mass in their spine while the group on the walking program gained 0.5 percent of bone mass (*AJCN.* 53:1304, 1991).

We suggest that people get in 10,000 steps every day. How you achieve those steps is up to you—simply do it *every* day. One way of achieving this goal is to invest in a pedometer or fitness tracker that you wear all day. It is a great motivational system for achieving a good level of activity throughout the day. A pedometer or any similar type tool for that matter that will increase weight-bearing activity will have a positive impact on bone health. However, it should be noted that this is just the diving board into a fit life. You must take it to the next level, which I call the X-factor.

The X-Factor in Bone Building

This is a very important section because it will describe to you the factor that will multiply your results many times over. Whenever we are discussing exercise, it is important to realize that there are three main factors to consider: volume, load, and intensity. Volume has to do with the number of repetitions. For walking the volume is high because you are repeating the movement over and over with only the load of your body for weight. This is, therefore, considered a high volume, low-load, low-intensity activity.

Load refers to the amount of weight involved in the activity. For our discussion, a small load is considered any weight that is easy to move, and a higher load is anything that is heavier than your body is used to moving. Doing a squat (sitting and standing motion) that allows you to complete only 6 to 8 repetitions is considered a high-load activity, provided that you cannot do the ninth repetition without assistance. Finally, intensity has to do with the rate and force in which you are performing the activity. Walking would be considered low intensity while sprinting is high intensity.

High-intensity activity usually results in a more percussive force, such as a heel strike on the road during sprinting. This results in a significantly increased load to the body.

Enough with the fitness jargon already. What is the significance of it all? Although it is common for healthcare providers to suggest weight-bearing activity, such as walking, as all that is necessary to improve bones, it will not be sufficient to optimize gains in bone density and quality. For the most part, walking will help to slow down bone loss but will do little to promote new bone formation, unless you previously have been confined to a bed or chair. However, we can add an X-factor to a simple walking program by increasing the load with a weighted vest. By adding a weighted vest, you increase the load on the bones by between 10 to 60 pounds. With that said, most of you will probably max out between 10 to 20 pounds, but do not let me limit you. The key is not to overdo the load, especially for high-volume activities, such as walking. If you add 5 pounds and that feels like a heavy load, then that is the weight you will use for now. Just be sure to increase the load as that weight becomes easier.

I fully expect you to have to shorten the volume of your walking due to fatigue. That is to be expected and even welcomed because load and intensity will always outperform volume as it pertains to the bones. If you increase the load and can walk for only 10 minutes compared with an hour without the weight, then so be it. Your bones will benefit all the more. With time, that 10 minutes will turn to 15 and then 20 and so on.

With bone health, the higher the load and intensity, the healthier your bones will become. Weight lifting is far more impactful in helping to maintain a healthy skeleton. If you are new to weightlifting, setting up a couple of sessions with a personal trainer is a good investment. During your time with the trainer, do not simply rely on him/her to train you, *Learn how to train yourself.* If you have osteoporosis, you may need the assistance of a physical therapist to teach you which exercises you can and cannot do. This would be a worthy investment in your health.

I commonly suggest that my clients become "fitness stars." What I mean by that is that you immerse yourself in a healthy lifestyle. People should be able to look at you and see energy and vitality. They should be able to realize that you know all about fitness by the way you are always reading new books and magazines and constantly talking about fitness. To me, fitness is the study of maintaining a youthful body that includes your bones.

I like to tell a story of a traveler in ancient Greece who was looking for Mount Olympus when he came upon a wise old man at a fork in the road. The young traveler inquired of the old man, "How do I get to Mount Olympus?" The wise old man, who happened to be Socrates, replied, "Just make sure that every step you take is in the direction of Mount Olympus." When you are trying to build strong bones, there is no neutral ground; your bones are either growing or diminishing. Just make sure that everything you do, every step you take is in the direction of strong bones.

A common question: "Exactly how much exercise is necessary to build bones?" The first answer is "the more, the better," which applies to conventional forms of resistance training. It is really difficult to get too much exercise in relation to improving bone density. There are instances where young women athletes have overtrained their way into osteoporosis, but this occurs only with women who train aggressively *and* are malnourished for the level of activity that they are taking part in. Remember, weight lifting does not make you fit; it only offers you the potential to get stronger and more fit. The strength and fitness come while you rest and rebuild. In order to make sure that you repair and regenerate properly after exercise, you must keep well nourished, with plenty of protein and natural, unrefined carbohydrates.

To give you a more objective answer to the question, we will turn to the scientific literature. In one study, women who partook in vigorous activity twice a week or more often or totaled 4 hours of physical activity a week had significantly greater bone density than women with a less aggressive exercise program. This study speaks to prevention. But what if you have significant bone loss? It seems that two weekly sessions of vigorous exercise are the minimum requirement for improving bone density. In postmenopausal women, high-intensity strength training performed twice a week yielded significant increases in bone density. However, increasing the aggressiveness of the workout schedule results in even further increases.

A study performed at the University of Washington in Saint Louis by Gail Dalsky, PhD, showed that an aggressive exercise program can significantly improve bone density in postmenopausal women. Both aerobic activity and strength training were performed in three weekly sessions of 50 to 60 minutes. The subjects also received a modest nutritional supplement with 1,500 mg of calcium and vitamin D. The results were astounding: after nine months, the postmenopausal women gained 5.2 percent in spinal mineral density. After 22 months. the women had gained 6.1 percent in bone density. Keep in mind, these women were expected to lose bone density in this time period (*Ann Intern Med.* 108.6;824–828; 1988).

In one study, researchers examined the effect of exercise in three groups of postmenopausal women: One group did no exercise, the second group did 30 minutes of aerobic activity at 80 percent of their maximum heart rate (a vigorous activity that likely exposed their body to significant force), and the third group added 10 to 15 minutes of mild strength training to the aerobic program. After one year, the group who performed no exercise had lost bone density, the group that did aerobic exercise increased bone density by 4.1 percent; and the group that did aerobic exercise and mild strength training increased their bone density by a whopping 7.5 percent (*BMJ.* 295; 231–234; 1987).

Degree of strain on the bones may be even *more* important than time spent exercising when it comes to bone density. One British study found that women who simply jump up and down 50 times a day can actually increase bone density and decrease the risk of fracture. Please note that this is not an exercise for people with osteoporosis, but it would be a good daily drill for young women who are not osteoporotic.

Experiment on Weight Lifting and Bones

In a well-controlled and fascinating study, researchers compared a weight-lifting routine that involves high-load and low-repetition (6 to 8 repetitions) with one that involved low-load and high-reps (20 reps). Each of the participants exercised only one side of the body, which allowed each person to act as their own control subject. The study results showed that the high-load, low-rep program resulted in a significant increase in bone density, while the low-load, high-rep program was ineffective. In addition, it was noted that the exercised limb showed significant improvement in bone density while the nonexercised side declined (*J Bone Miner Res.* 1996:11:218–225).

Warning:

Exercise is wonderful for building bones, but exercising too much with insufficient rest can cause a bone breakdown. This is usually only a concern with elite athletes who stress their bodies beyond design specs and do not get enough good-quality nutrition. People who sweat profusely may be at greater risk for mineral deficiencies that can place them at risk for osteoporosis. Cyclists have a tendency to have very low bone density because they sweat out important minerals and the activity is not weight bearing or strength promoting. Cyclists should be on a regular strength-training program and get higher doses of calcium, magnesium, and other trace minerals.

Top Recommendations for Exercising to Build Bones!

1. Exercise at least twice weekly (3 times weekly for best results).
2. If you are not at risk of bone fracture, make your exercise as vigorous as

you can tolerate. Be sure that you get guidance if you are unsure of how aggressive you can be.

3. For aerobic activity, try to work up to 70 to 80 percent of your maximum heart rate for 20 to 30 minutes to stimulate the most bone development. You can figure your maximum heart rate by subtracting your age from 220; to figure 70 percent of the maximum heart rate simply multiply the number you get by 0.7. (Example: 50-year-old woman. $220 - 50 = 170 * 0.7 = 119$.) It is not the increase in heart rate that offers the benefit to the bone, but rather the impact of each stride.

4. When strength-training, it is best to do one good set of 8 to 10 different exercises that stress different muscles (*Medicine & Science in Sports & Exercise.* 32(1): 235–242, 2000). A person can achieve a great strength-training workout in 20 to 30 minutes.

5. Aim for a weight that allows you to do only 6 to 8 repetitions. If you can do the ninth repetition, then increase

the weight slightly so that you are working in the 6- to 8-repetition range.

6. Start by working with a lighter weight that allows you to perform 15 to 20 repetitions. As you get stronger, increase the weight you lift while decreasing the repetitions. Small changes are all that is necessary to facilitate change.

7. Never replace good exercise technique with more weight.

8. Achieve 10,000 steps *every* day. Use a pedometer or fitness tracker.

9. Work out with a partner; motivate each other to stick with the program.

10. Never exercise hungry. Have a snack or meal 2 or 3 hours before your workout. Have a protein shake soon after the workout to improve the ability of the muscle to repair and rebuild (SlimFast® or Ensure® do not cut it).

11. Get plenty of sleep. Exercise breaks the body down, while rest and sleep rebuild the body. Sleep promotes the production of anabolic hormones,

such as growth hormones, which promote bone growth.

12. Never exercise the same muscle group two days in a row. Do not exercise a muscle that still hurts from the previous workout; this is a sign that tissue repair is not complete.

13. When starting a program, expect discomfort for a few days after the workout. This will subside, and after continued workouts, you will find that your muscles will no longer ache after workouts.

14. Use a weighted vest whenever you go for a walk. You may also want to purchase a pair of walking poles, similar to ski poles, to help prevent falls.

15. Never do exercises that cause you to bend the spine in awkward positions, such as crunches, sit-ups, and ball exercises.

16. The number one cause of fractures is falling. Performing exercises that promote balance can significantly decrease the risk of fracture by keeping you on your feet.

Vibration for Stronger Bones

In recent years, a machine known as a Whole Body Vibration Plate has been receiving press for its ability to reverse osteoporosis. This machine requires a person to simply stand on the machine in a semisquat position while the machine vibrates up and down at a fairly rapid rate. This vibration forces the fast-twitch muscles to contract rapidly, which applies stress to the bones and forces them to grow stronger. The manufacturers make a number of interesting claims, such as:

- Extremely safe for osteoporosis.
- If you can stand, then you can do it.
- Increases strength.
- Improves balance.
- Takes 10 to 12 minutes 3 to 7 days a week.
- Improves flexibility.
- Improves circulation.

Are These Claims True?

From the research that I can gather, it appears that these claims *are* at least partially true. One study took two groups of postmenopausal women and put them on two different routines to evaluate the effect on bone density. One group received three sessions per week of whole-body vibration, with each session being six sets of 1 minute of whole-body vibration followed by 1 minute of rest. This amounted to a total workout time of 11 minutes per session. The second group was placed on a walking routine of 55 minutes three times a week. After eight months, the group receiving whole-body vibration enjoyed a 4.3 percent increase in bone mineral density of the leg bone and a 29 percent improvement in balance; the walking group showed little improvement. Unfortunately, there was no significant change in bone density of the spine in any either group (*BMC Musculoskelet Disord.* 2006 Nov 30;7:92).

In another study, researchers had one group of postmenopausal, osteoporotic women perform one 10-minute session of whole-body vibration five days a week for six months. The control group made no change to their lifestyle. The results were astounding: After three months of whole-body vibration, the lumbar spine had improved in density by 1.3 percent, and after six months there was a 4.3 percent increase in lumbar spine density. The control group lost bone density in the lumbar spine by the sixth month. The whole-body vibration group improved the density of their leg bone (femur) by 3.2 percent after six months. The control group lost bone density by the study's end. Back pain improved in the group receiving whole-body vibration.

So it does appear that whole-body vibration can be an alternative to conventional exercise, especially in people who are unable to do resistance training because of injury or arthritis. In addition, whole-body vibration appears to improve balance, which could protect you from unnecessary falls.

Two Types of Vibration Therapy

There are two types of vibration therapy: high-intensity vibration therapy and low-intensity vibration (LIV) therapy. The high-intensity vibration plates are often found in gyms and commonly used by athletes. These plates are much more expensive and are less appropriate for frail seniors who can be injured if the machines are used inappropriately. The low-intensity vibration therapy is considered safe and effective for people who are frail and those diagnosed with osteoporosis. In addition, the low-intensity vibration plates are more affordable and appropriate for daily home use. There are two manufacturers who produce well-researched platforms for home vibration therapy: Juvent (Juvent.com) and Marodyne LIV (https://marodyne.btt-health.com). Both are effective, although the Marodyne is more affordable. If you can afford one of these low-intensity vibration plates for home use, I highly recommend purchasing and using it daily.

Are There Any Contraindications to Vibration Treatment?

Low-intensify vibration is safe for most people. That being said, it is a good idea to always discuss your treatment plans with your doctor before starting any physical activity. There are situations when high-intensity vibration treatment should be avoided:

- Pregnancy
- Severe cardiovascular disease
- If you have a pacemaker
- If you have a seizure disorder
- If you suffer from severe migraines
- If you suffer from a deep vein thrombosis (DVT)
- If you have recently injured yourself
- If you have had recent surgery
- If you have had a knee or hip replacement
- If you have had a history of kidney stones (*J Sports Med Phys Fitness.* 2007;47:443–445)
- If you have a history or risk of retinal detachment

Final Notes On Vibration Therapy For Osteoporosis

Whole-body vibration can be an effective tool, and with more manufacturers producing these machines, the treatment is becoming more widely available. I recommend choosing one of the low-intensity vibration machines listed above. Please purchase only a high-quality machine in order to prevent injury. These low-intensity machines—which cost between $2,500 and $5,000—are very easy to use. Simply stand on them for 10 minutes per day, and you are done. Research suggests that there are a number of positive benefits beyond stronger bones These machines can also help to improve circulation, to decrease pain, and to improve healing after surgery.

How To Reverse Osteoporosis In Just 7-Minutes A Week

In my experience, it has been frustratingly difficult to get many of my patients to put in the time and effort in the gym to build their bones and to reverse osteoporosis. The fact is, exercising with sufficient load and intensity is difficult and time-consuming. I have had great difficulty getting my own mother to exercise beyond just walking and swimming, especially given her asthma that limits the amount of effort she can exert during exercise.

I am happy to report that there is a new technology called BioDensity that is becoming more and more popular. The BioDensity machine is a patented piece of high-tech exercise equipment that allows someone to exercise just 7 minutes a week without discomfort and in such a safe manner that it can be used by people with DXA scores as low as -4.0. The best part is, with just 7 minutes of exercise performed once a week, you can actually see dramatic increases in bone density within one year. Many people who have trained with BioDensity equipment have reported better results than people who are working out in the gym for an hour three to five days a week. It sounds too good to be true, but early research is confirming the effectiveness and safety of the BioDensity. The manufacturer claims that the average increase in bone density from clients who have used the machine once weekly in centers across the country is 4 to 7 percent. These numbers are unheard of and, if confirmed over the next few years, would equate to a breakthrough in osteoporosis treatment.

One study, published in the journal *Osteoporosis International,* evaluated the use of the BioDensity machine in 15 postmenopausal women between ages 56 and 84. The women in the study trained once a week on the BioDensity machine, with each session lasting just 15 minutes, start to finish. After one year, 11 of the 15 enjoyed an increase in bone density, 2 had no bone loss, and only 2 of the 15 showed worsening of bone density (*Osteoporosis International.* Vol. 29, Supplement 1, April 2018.).

Another study presented the results of the BioDensity on 14 men and women who used the machine once per week for approximately one year, with the results presented in case-study format. After one year, the average increase in bone density was 7.02 percent in the hips and 7.73 percent in the spine (*Osteoporosis International*, 198 Volume 24, Supplement 4, December [2013] S594–S595).

Another study evaluated the side benefits of the BioDensity in subjects between ages 85 and 93. Not surprisingly, the subjects who performed 5 minutes of exercise on the BioDensity experienced improvements in strength between 22 to 51 percent. In addition, they improved in all measured functions of daily living, including the ability to ascend and descend stairs, walking speed, walking distance, ability to stand from a seated position, and balance.

The company that manufactures the BioDensity machine continues to run aftermarket research on it through voluntary submission of DXA scans from many current users of the technology. Regular users of the BioDensity also report significant improvements in strength in as little as one week, a better range of motion, fewer aches and pains, and even improvements in blood sugar in diabetic patients.

Now the bad news: BioDensity is not yet available in many areas. If you are in the Baltimore/Owings Mills area of Maryland, visit us at OsteoCoach.com for details about training on the BioDensity machine. For the rest of you in other states and countries, visit BioDensity.com to see if there is a center in your area that provides the service. If there is no place available, stay tuned as I expect the BioDensity machine to become the gold-standard mechanical treatment for osteoporosis in the future.

One final note, although the BioDensity may trigger more bone remodeling than any other form of exercise, you should make it part of a comprehensive fitness program that includes other forms of resistance training and walking.

Soapbox Comments Regarding Exercise & Activity

I cannot do justice to the importance of exercise and activity for promoting strong bones for life. To sum up the importance of exercise, I would say this, "If you do one thing in this program, and one thing only, it would be exercise." I have too many patients who have no problem popping a few pills but continue to live a sedentary life, and their bone density suffers for it. Supplements simply are not enough. It is my intention to help as many people as I can to live active lives without the worry of breaking a bone or losing their lives to osteoporosis-related causes. I realize, after reviewing the research literature, that exercise is a major piece of the puzzle. Please, decide today to get up and live an active lifestyle. Your skeleton is depending on it!

14

The Perfect Bone-Building Diet

Introduction to the Diet-Bone Connection

Every year or two, every molecule in your body is completely turned over. This means that every year or two you are literally a completely new person made up of entirely new cells. Your bones are no different. I think that many people mistakenly view the bones as a structure similar to limestone with no life, no dynamics. In fact, we have already learned that bones are constantly being broken down and regenerated every moment that we are alive.

So what will you be made of one to two years from now?

Remember, the food that you take in today will become the brick and mortar of your cells tomorrow. Will you be made up of soft, gooey bonbons and milkshakes? Or energetic fruits, vegetables, nuts, seeds, and lean proteins? It is your choice …

Science has found that bones prefer to be made up of certain foods. It is no secret that a bone-building diet is comprised of high quantities of vegetables, fruits, nuts, and seeds. I realize, however, that most people do not want to live their lives as vegetarians. In fact, I feel that you can achieve a healthy skeleton even if meat comprises a significant part of your diet. Below, I will describe 10 steps that will help your bones grow stronger with time.

10 Point Bone-Building Diet

POINT 1: Eat 3 times more vegetables, nuts, and seeds than meat or refined carbohydrates.

Green, leafy vegetables—such as collard greens, kale, mustard greens, baby greens, parsley, and escarole—are all great sources of calcium, magnesium, vitamin K, and folic acid. Some greens—such as spinach, chard, and beet greens—can have high levels of oxalate that may bind and prevent the absorption of calcium, so they should be eaten in smaller quantities. Overall, I believe that oxalate-containing greens are not harmful; they just may not provide the extra kick to bone development that the previously mentioned greens would. Greens also help to maintain an optimum calcium/phosphorus balance.

POINT 2: Stop the soda madness.

Soda is a source of phosphates that throws off the delicate calcium/phosphate balance of the body, resulting in a significant decrease in blood calcium levels. In fact, there appears to be an inverse relationship between the number of bottles of soda consumed and the blood levels of calcium. This means that the more soda you drink, the lower your blood calcium levels will be (*J Adolesc Health.* 1994;15:210–215). To replace that calcium in the blood, the body will be forced to withdraw it from your bones. Soda is a huge negative mark against your bones, so avoid drinking it. More importantly, keep your kids away from it. Sparkling water can be used in place of soda, but good old-fashioned water is best.

POINT 3: Limit sugar and refined carbohydrates to an absolute minimum.

Refined carbohydrates and sugar cause a significant loss of calcium from the body. Try to limit these products, such as white bread, pasta, white rice, cakes, candy, sugar, etc. (*Br J Urol.* 1978;50:459–464).

A study examining rats demonstrated the importance of controlling sugar intake. In this study, two groups of rats were fed similar diets. The only difference between the groups was that one received sugar as its primary carbohydrate and the other group received a slower-absorbing starch. At the end of the study, it was discovered that the bones of rats whose diet contained sucrose (table sugar) as its carbohydrate source broke much easier than the bones of the group given the same amount of carbohydrate in the form of starch (*J Nutri.* 128(10):1807–1810).

POINT 4: Limit sodium intake.

Sodium is found in unnaturally high levels in our diet. Sodium has been shown to cause calcium loss when it is in excess. Allow me to provide you with a secret that may make your life a little easier: it is okay to sprinkle salt on your food. The majority of your sodium intake comes from prepared and processed food rather than from table salt. Pay more attention to the canned, boxed, and prepared foods, as they are your biggest sodium supplier. There is evidence that gray sea salt is far superior to standard table salt as a means of seasoning your food. Sea salt has a little less sodium and more trace minerals, which may provide additional benefits. Potassium and sodium are a couple of peas in the same pod, and there is evidence that eating foods with higher potassium levels may take some of the stings out of the high sodium levels in our diet. It would be optimal to decrease sodium intake while simultaneously increasing potassium intake. Another alternative to standard table salt is a formula called GoodSalt which uses potassium and magnesium in place of sodium.

Although excess sodium should be avoided; it is equally devastating to consume too little sodium. Sodium is an essential component of normal metabolism, and without sufficient sodium, many systems—such as the nervous, digestive, and skeletal systems—cannot function properly. I see many more people whose sodium intake falls on either side of the extremes, consuming either way too much or way too little sodium. Look for the balance. If in doubt, it is better to consume slightly too much, rather than slightly too little, as the body has the ability to excrete modest excesses of sodium. If you follow Point 1, eating three times more plants than refined food, you will get a healthy dose of potassium to counteract excess sodium.

POINT 5: Get the healthy omega-3 fatty acids from diet and supplements.

Omega-3 fatty acids are very important for maintaining bone structure. Foods such as cold-water fish, sardines, nuts, and seeds contain good levels of polyunsaturated fatty acids. For those of you who do not like to eat fish, then be sure to take extra care to add omega-3 fats from fish sources (such as salmon, sardines, and tuna). If you are vegetarian, you can add omega-3 fats from flaxseed, salba seed, or hemp seed. If you choose the vegetarian source, then make sure that you add 200 to 400 mg of DHA from an algae source (found in health-food stores under the Neuromins brand).

POINT 6: Get plenty of fresh, clean water.

Water is very important for maintaining a healthy pH of the blood. The body will steal calcium from the bones if the pH is not properly maintained. I recommend 60 to 80 ounces per day.

POINT 7: Eat mostly lean proteins.

Protein intake, as it pertains to bone density, has been the subject of great debate for some time because the studies have been inconsistent. The Nurses' Health Study found that the nurses who had a higher intake of animal protein also had a higher risk of forearm fracture; the nurses who had more vegetarian sources of protein did not suffer the same risk. It is hypothesized that meat is an acid-producing food and thus can put a lot of strain on the mineral bank account of bones. Studies that compare vegetarians with omnivores found that bone mineral density is not significantly different up until the fifth decade. After that, omnivores have significantly lower bone densities.

On the flip side, the Framingham Osteoporosis Study evaluated the habits of 543 people (319 women and 224 men) between ages 69 and 91. They discovered that study subjects with the lowest protein intake were at increased risk of bone fracture compared with those with the highest protein intake. The individuals whose protein intake was in the lowest 25 percent suffered 50 percent more hip fractures. According to this study, the researchers recommend consuming a daily minimum of 46 gm of protein for women and 56 gm of protein for men (*Osteoporosis International*, May 2010). Another study conducted at Tufts University found that people who ate high protein and low carbohydrates actually had decreased calcium loss and increased bone growth factors in their blood.

So what should you do?

Judging from an analysis of all the data, moderate protein consumption is unlikely to negatively impact bones, provided you decrease the number of refined carbohydrates and increase the amount of alkalinizing fruits and vegetables. For overall bone health, I recommend consuming three servings of vegetables for every serving of animal protein that you consume daily. It should be noted that vegetarian protein, such as fermented soy, does not appear to cause the same potential problems as animal protein. There is strong evidence that alkalinizing diets— lower in protein and higher in vegetation—can be a very important factor in the fight against osteoporosis. For this reason, I wrote an additional chapter titled "The pH Factor." For now, whenever you consume protein, you should also enjoy a big salad to counteract the acid found in the meat. It is also recommended that you consume fewer refined carbohydrates throughout the day. After you have read "The pH Factor," you can further tweak your program.

POINT 8: Limit Dairy.

We already covered this subject in a previous section. Just know that milk is food for calves, not for humans. Dairy is not a natural food for us, and a number of studies have linked dairy consumption to increased fracture risk. You can build healthy bones without consuming large amounts of dairy. The bottom line on dairy, as it pertains to bones, is it is not the bone-building miracle it is made out to be. Do not expect dairy to protect your bones from osteoporosis.

POINT 9: Limit coffee intake.

Caffeine from coffee, but not tea, appears to increase urinary excretion of calcium and possibly other minerals from the body. One or 2 cups daily are probably safe and even healthy However, if you are osteoporotic, I would recommend avoiding large quantities of caffeinated coffee. I have met people who drink an entire pot of coffee per day, but limiting it to 2 cups or fewer per day is advised (1 standard cup of coffee is approximately 8 ounces).

POINT 10: Limit alcohol intake.

Alcohol is another one of those compounds that causes calcium to be leached from the body. Alcohol is a double-edged sword, with overall health and the bones no different. It appears that moderate alcohol intake provides some modest protection for osteoporosis, possibly due to a slight increase in estrogen and calcitonin production. Intake of greater than 7 ounces of alcohol weekly has been shown to increase your risk of falls and fracture, so be careful (*Calcif Tissue Int.* 1991;49(supp):S70–73). Stick to no more than one serving of alcohol per day. If you have a tendency to drink too much, it is imperative that you fix this part of your lifestyle, as it can negate many of the benefits of an otherwise healthy lifestyle.

Water – The Missing Component

In the television comedy "Seinfeld," Jerry walks up to get the rental car he had reserved days before when the representative tells him, "We are all out of vehicles." Jerry, dumbfounded by the announcement, questions the young lady behind the counter, saying, "But I have a reservation." She again says, "I am so sorry, but we are out of cars." Jerry, now a little frustrated says, "But the purpose of a reservation is to reserve a car so that you do not run out of cars for the customer!" She replies, "I know what a reservation is for...." He then responds, "I don't think you do! Because if you did, *I would have a car!*" Now, let me get to my point: many of you may feel like skipping this section because you already know about the importance of drinking water. I venture to say, "I don't think you do because if you did, *you would be drinking more water!*" Am I right?

Did you know that water makes up a whopping 25 percent of bone weight? Much like a desiccated tree snaps in the wind, bones become weak as they become depleted of vital water. Studies on the content of bones have determined that water fills the spaces between protein strands that hold your bones together. This water is believed to allow the bones to flex with movement, much like trees arch or bend when a stiff wind strikes them. Water is also essential to balancing pH and delivering vital minerals and nutrients to bones. So grab a bottle and sip on water all day long. (While you are at it, give up the sodas!)

Are Your Chocolate Days Over?

When I saw the headline "Chocolate Causes Osteoporosis," I knew I was in trouble. As expected, I came into the office to tons of emails from chocolate lovers everywhere who wanted to know if their love affair with their creamy sweetie was at an end. It especially hit home when my own mother told me that she was giving up her occasional dark chocolate square because she read the news that her bones were damned if she did not cease consuming chocolate entirely.

So What Is the deal?

In a recent study, scientists evaluated the food diaries of over 1,000 senior women ages 70 to 85. After assessing the records and comparing a number of variables with bone density, it was discovered that women who ate chocolate one or more times daily had weaker bones than those who ate it less than once a week. In fact, the group who ate chocolate daily had bone densities that were 3.1 percent lower than their counterparts who ate chocolate less than once per week.

Thus, the headline "Chocolate Causes Osteoporosis."

So does chocolate really cause osteoporosis? Not likely. This study is considered preliminary research because it does not show cause and effect. Although the statistics indicate a correlation between chocolate and bone loss, there are just too many other factors (perhaps thousands) that can account for the findings that chocolate eaters have lower bone density. For instance, is it possible that people who eat chocolate daily take less care of themselves compared with people who eat it once a week? In my book, daily chocolate consumption suggests either a lack of health knowledge or a disregard for health and fitness. Is it then feasible that the group who eats chocolate daily also eats other acidic and/or sugary foods, drinks more sodas, exercises less, etc.?

Of course! This study falls into a class of research called observational or epidemiological research, which is considered the weakest form of study. This type of research commonly acts as the launching board for more expensive and involved double-blind research. However, in the case of chocolate, I doubt we will see this type of research completed.

Is it possible that these findings are accurate? Is it possible that there is some compound in chocolate that causes bone loss? As a scientist, I must concede the possibility, but it is *highly* unlikely. Should we eat chocolate daily? Of course not, at least not in quantity But should my dear mother—who eats well, takes her supplements, and goes to her daily "Guts and Butts" exercise class—avoid her chocolate square once or twice a week? No! She is 83 years young and deserves to enjoy her chocolate square. It is just unfortunate that many people will likely fall prey to this danger ploy so that others can sell newspapers.

As a side note, there is also a difference between dark chocolate and milk chocolate. Dark chocolate is very low in sugar and high in antioxidants that may be quite healthy for the bones and body. A The average milk chocolate "candy bar"of milk chocolate is high in sugar and devoid of significant antioxidants. A However, a couple of squares of dark chocolate daily are likely to be perfectly healthy.

Does Soy Do a Body Good?

In many small-scale studies, soy isoflavones have been shown to decrease bone loss and to increase bone formation. However, due to the small number of people in each of the studies, it is difficult to accept the results until larger-scale studies of a similar nature have been completed. In the absence of these larger studies, researchers attempt to combine numerous small studies into what is called a meta-analysis to look for significant results that may give more support to the results in question. Two such meta-analysis studies were published in two separate peer-reviewed studies that may shed some light on the true significance of soy studies.

The first study involved 432 perimenopausal and postmenopausal women who either consumed soy protein or soy tablets containing high amounts of soy isoflavones for between 4 to 48 weeks. The scientists measured urinary markers of bone loss, as well as serum markers of bone formation. After evaluating all of the data, they concluded that "isoflavone intervention significantly inhibits bone resorption [loss] and stimulates bone formation [repair and growth]" (*Eur J Clin Nutr.* 2008 Feb;62:155–61).

In the second study, researchers evaluated studies that totaled 608 perimenopausal and postmenopausal women who ate high levels of soy protein or soy isoflavone supplements for 3 to 48 months. The results were most significant for postmenopausal women and showed significant increases in spinal bone density (*Clin Nutr.* 2008 Feb;27(1):57-64).

Both of these meta-analysis studies should open the door for larger-scale studies on soy isoflavones. Due to the small-scale nature of the studies to date, I have not made soy a significant part of my program in *Strong Bones Forever.* With this data, I feel that some women may find soy a useful tool in their program. Currently, I recommend that women limit their intake of soy isoflavones to 50 mg daily from food and supplements. Fermented soy products are considered best as they more most closely mimic the diet of Asian cultures, which have been linked to stronger bones and lower risks of breast cancer.

What is Ipriflavone? Is It Effective for Osteoporosis? Is It Safe?

Ipriflavone is a synthetic isoflavone similar to the plant estrogens found in soy and other herbs. Given that ipriflavone is synthetic; I consider it to be more of a drug than a nutritional supplement.

Ipriflavone Benefits

The evidence to date of the benefits of taking ipriflavone has been inconclusive; some studies suggest an improvement in bone density, while more recent and better-controlled studies have shown no significant difference between ipriflavone and placebo. Even if we were to give ipriflavone the benefit of the doubt and accept it as an effective tool in increasing the density of bones, I would still be hesitant to recommend it to my patients. When we look at the mechanism by which isoflavones (such as ipriflavone) as a class work on the bones, you will note that it is not unlike the medications that I rally against. Isoflavones work by inhibiting the breakdown of old, brittle bone. As I teach you in the book, this process (called bone resorption) is a necessary process if your goal is to build healthy, strong bone. We want to build new, strong, pliable bone rather than just maintain the density by keeping around old, brittle bone. The research on ipriflavone is simply not strong enough to warrant the "Osteoporosis Diet Stamp of Approval."

Ipriflavone Side Effects:

I wish I could say that the ipriflavone drug (yes, I consider it a drug) is, at worst, ineffective. Unfortunately, studies have drawn the safety of this drug into question. In studies, patients who were taking the ipriflavone showed a decreased number of disease-fighting white blood cells. In my practice, I have witnessed this effect in patients who came to my office already taking ipriflavone. This means that ipriflavone could decrease your ability to fight viruses, bacteria, and cancer.

Ipriflavone appears to inhibit certain enzymes in the liver, which could lead to an interaction with certain medications that are metabolized through the cytochrome p450 pathway. Although there are few published cases of such an interaction with ipriflavone, caution should be exercised when using it with other medications.

Ipriflavone is considered a drug because it is a synthetic compound, and there is no such thing as a natural ipriflavone source. In addition, the product has a mechanism of action and side effects that make it resemble a drug rather than a nutritional ingredient. Needless to say, this product gets a thumbs-down from me.

What About Antioxidants?

Years ago, scientists discovered that certain compounds in the body, called free radicals, could damage tissues and lead to premature aging.

These free radicals are formed through normal metabolism; however, it was also discovered that certain environmental and lifestyle situations could also contribute to the production of these unstable oxidants. The increased production of free radicals is hypothesized to speed the aging process. In fact, there is plenty of evidence to suggest that these free radicals do contribute to the aging process.

Free radicals, it turns out, are not all bad. As I mentioned, free radicals are produced during normal metabolism. In addition, immune cells use free radicals as a weapon against unwanted invaders. Luckily, Mother Nature, realizing the potential harm that these free radicals can cause, gave us compounds, called antioxidants, that help to protect the healthy cells from damage. Antioxidants are abundant in nature, found in high levels in many fruits, vegetables, nuts, and seeds. These compounds exist in practically every cell of the body and are constantly standing guard against excess levels of free radicals in the body.

So what does this have to do with bones? Well, it turns out that the cells of bones are not immune from free radicals, and recent research has shown that a healthy supply of antioxidants is critical to the proper function of bone-building cells.

In one study, a form of vitamin E called gamma tocotrienols improved bone structure and strength (*J Bone Miner Metab.* 2009 September). In fact, this is not the first time that tocotrienols have proven themselves useful in the fight against osteoporosis. Another study found that tocotrienols could decrease inflammation in the bones that lead to bone loss.

Consuming lots of antioxidants in the diet is a good idea for bone health as well as health in general. I am not ready to recommend large quantities of supplemental antioxidants, such as vitamin C or E, but the good news is if you follow the recommendations in this chapter, you will be consuming an antioxidant-rich diet/

Chapter Summary:

In this chapter we discussed ten ways to improve your diet in favor of a healthy skeleton. These concepts include: 1. Eat three times more vegetables, nuts, and seeds than meat or refined carbohydrates. 2. Stop the soda. 3. Limit sugar and refined carbohydrates 4. Limit sodium intake. 5. Consume healthy omega-3 fatty acids from nuts, seeds, seafood, and supplements. 6. Drink lots of water. 7. Eat mostly lean protein. 8. Don't expect dairy to do all the work in building healthy bones 9. Limit coffee to two cups or less per day. 10 . Limit alcohol intake. All of these points are relatively easy to implement, but do not let their simplicity lull you into believing they are insignificant.

15

The pH Factor

Osteoporosis occurs when the bones are broken down faster than they are built up. If you read the previous chapters, then you should already understand this point. In this chapter, we are going to discuss how the pH balance of your body plays a major role in the health of your skeleton and how to correct the acid/base imbalance that is eroding your bone minerals with each passing second.

Bones act as more than just structural support for the body; they also act as a source of minerals and other compounds to buffer the blood in order to keep it from becoming too acidic. Should the blood become acidic (a process called metabolic acidosis), then the electrical activity of the body would become unstable, which could result in death. In order to prevent such a situation, the body responds by pulling minerals from the bone bank account to buffer the blood. This saves your life in the present, but damns you to osteoporosis if left unchecked. In order to successfully treat osteoporosis, we must prevent the eroding process by making sure that the body remains slightly alkaline without the need to dip into the skeleton for minerals and buffering agents.

To assess the effect of pH on bone cells, researchers performed an interesting study where they placed live bone tissue in a test tube environment and lowered pH (made more acidic) by just one-tenth of a point. This resulted in a significant increase in osteoclastic activity, which eats away at your bone mass, a significant decrease in the activity of the bone-building cells, and a multifold increase in bone mineral loss (*Am J Physiol.* 31:F442–F448,1992). In another study, a 0.2-point drop in pH resulted in a 500 to 900 percent increase in the activity of the cells, which break down bone and remove minerals (*Endocrinology.* 119:119–124,1986). These test tube results were confirmed in humans when the human subjects were placed in a fasting state that resulted in a blood pH change from 7.37 to 7.33, a change of 0.04 pH points.

As you can see, when the body's pH is even mildly altered, there is a significant increase in the bone breakdown, which can ultimately lead to osteoporosis if left unchecked.

In order to sustain life, the body must maintain a slightly alkaline pH. It has been demonstrated that blood from an artery should remain at a pH of between 7.35 and 7.45. This means that the healthy range of pH in the blood needs to remain at 7.4, give or take 0.5 pH points. If the blood falls outside this range, even by a tiny bit, it can have a catastrophic effect.

When we look inside a cell, the pH needs to remain under even tighter control; deviation of more than 0.1 point causes catastrophic results to occur. Such complications that can occur when intracellular pH of the blood becomes even slightly acidic include:

1. A decrease in energy formation in the cells
2. Poor metabolism
3. Decrease protein synthesis (repair and regeneration of the body)
4. Accelerated bone loss
5. More fluid retention
6. Hormonal imbalances

During normal metabolism, huge quantities of acid are produced; however, the body's own buffering systems work around the clock to sequester the acid and to maintain balance. More or less, acid can be liberated into the system depending on diet and lifestyle.

What Causes Excess Acid Load?

So far, scientists have discovered a number of diet and lifestyle factors that can result in excess acid load in the body. Excess protein intake can potentially increase acid load through its metabolism. There are certain amino acids, found especially in animal protein, that can lead to excess acidity after the body metabolizes them. These amino acids include:

1. Aspartate
2. Glutamate
3. Cysteine
4. Cystine
5. Proline/hydroxyproline
6. Threonine
7. Serine

It has also been noted that long-chain fatty acids found in many animal proteins can also add to the body's acid load.

There are also many alkaline buffering compounds that are brought into the system through food metabolism, including potassium, magnesium, calcium, and other minerals from fruits, vegetables, and spices. It is also known that shorter-chained fatty acids, such as those found in many vegetarian sources, can help to buffer out excess acid.

Please note, the acidity of the food itself is not an important factor. What *is* important is the acid or alkaline residue after the food has been digested and metabolized. This means that a product, such as citrus fruit, which is outwardly acid, becomes alkaline to the body after it has been metabolized. This is called the acid or alkaline "ash" of food.

It is well known that bones are made up of calcium and magnesium; but it is lesser known that potassium and sodium are very important minerals found in the bones as well. In fact, potassium and sodium are loosely bound minerals in the bones, which make them readily accessible to the body during times of acidity.

During times of acidity, the body quickly dips into the potassium, sodium, and carbonate stores, which can be found ready for mobilization in the outer shell of bone. It is only after prolonged exposure to the acidity that the body begins to dip into the calcium and magnesium. Having evaluated the lab results of hundreds of patients, it is not uncommon to see less-than-optimal and even overtly low-sodium and/or potassium levels, especially in seniors. It is curious that this type of electrolyte imbalance is found in seniors, a group that is at greatest risk of osteoporotic fracture. Potassium is also a very common deficiency in the diet, due to a lack of fruits and vegetables.

Incidentally, diet is not the only factor that plays a role in pH balance. Stress is well known for changing the body's balance in such a way that it promotes acidity. This is likely due to the excess production of adrenaline and cortisol. It is also possible for food allergies—such as dairy, wheat, and gluten—to play a role in acidifying the body.

Another factor that needs to be discussed is the effect of carbonated drinks on acid load. It has been noted that soda has a pH between 2.8 and 3.2 (very acidic). In order to process that much acid, the kidneys would have to dilute one 12-ounce soda with 33 liters of water to bring the pH to a level that the urinary tract could tolerate. Obviously, this would not be possible, so the body must dip into the buffering agents of the bones to correct the pH and to balance the system again. It has been suggested that one soda would require the buffering capacity of four Tums to neutralize the acid in that single can of soda.

Follow these steps to improve the acid/alkaline balance:

1. Drink plenty of water. Water acts as the first defense against excess acid.
2. I recommend between 60 to 80 ounces of water daily. This is a lot of water, but this quantity can provide major benefits to the body that go well beyond the benefit to acid/alkaline balance. The color of the urine should be light yellow or completely clear.
3. Eat mostly raw fruits and vegetables that are full of alkaline minerals. Different fruits and vegetables provide different levels of acid-neutralizing benefits. See Appendix A for a report card of various foods for balancing pH.

4. Add 20 to 40 drops of ConcenTrace® Trace Mineral Drops, by Trace Mineral Research to each 32-ounce

bottle of water you drink to add trace minerals to the water to increase the alkalinizing effect of the water.

5. Whenever you eat animal protein, eat a big salad to balance out the acid.

6. Drink freshly pressed fruit and vegetable juices. This fresh juice will contain high levels of buffering minerals. A full 8 ounces daily adds a helpful buffer against the acid in the diet; some people with higher acidity may need more. If juicing is not feasible, then add an alkalinizing greens powder to your water. Visit OsteoCoach.com/StrongBonesForever for a list of quality green food powders.

7. Follow the recommendations in *Strong Bones Forever.*

8. Optional: Test your first-morning urine on a regular basis, using pH paper or strips. Shoot for a first-morning urine pH of 6.5 to 7.5.

9. Monitor your stress levels and learn coping mechanisms to control stress.

16

The Mind-Bone Connection

Depressed? The Bones Know…

Depression is emerging as an important risk factor in osteoporosis. We have always ascertained that every cell of our bodies is eavesdropping on our thoughts. This means that when we think a certain thought that causes a stress reaction, then the body kicks out a certain set of chemicals into the bloodstream that impacts each and every cell in the body. Said another way, when you think angry thoughts, a series of neurotransmitters and hormones are secreted into the brain and bloodstream, and you feel the emotion of anger. In addition to your mind feeling anger, these same neurotransmitters and hormones connect with the cells in your arteries, red blood cells, and bone cells—and, in a sense, these cells become angry as well.

Dozens of studies have demonstrated a direct connection to negative emotions and bone loss. One such study determined that depressed perimenopausal women suffered a 7.8 percent reduction in bone density compared with happier counterparts (*Menopause.* 2005 Jan-Feb;12(1): 88–91). Other studies have demonstrated that depression can result in between a 6 to 15 percent loss of bone compared with nondepressed people (*J Psychiatry.* 1994 Nov;151(11):1691–3; *N Engl J Med.* 1996 Oct 17;335(16):1176–81).

How does Depression Impact the Bones?

There are a number of theories as to how depression impacts the health of the skeleton. The likelihood is that all the current theories are at least partly to blame for the failing skeletons of depressed and chronically stressed individuals. Let us discuss some of these reasons ...

Behavioral factors: People who are depressed have a tendency to stay indoors (limits sun exposure), be sedentary, smoke more, eat poorly, and drink more alcohol. As we have already discussed, all of these factors negatively impact the formation of bone.

More medications: Depressed individuals may be more likely to be on medications that predispose them for osteoporosis. An example would be medications used to treat heartburn and ulcers, which are both more common in depressed patients. They may also be more likely to be on drugs, such as benzodiazepines, that make them unsteady on their feet, thus placing them at higher risk of falls.

Depression and stress cause excess production of stress hormones: Cortisol is secreted during stress and can result in bone loss. People who are depressed likely secrete more cortisol, which can erode bone over time.

Depression increases inflammation: Studies have shown that depression increases the secretion of inflammatory chemicals, which are known to negatively impact bone. One such compound is Interleukin 6, which stimulates bone breakdown.

Depression can cause deficiency of anabolic hormones: Growth hormone and testosterone can become deficient in people who are afflicted with chronic depression. Both of these hormones are extremely important in keeping the skeleton healthy.

Depression and anxiety can go hand in hand: Often people will suffer from both depression and anxiety, leading to medications, such as benzodiazepines, which are linked to a significantly increased risk of falls and fractures.

So What Do We Do About It?

The first thing to do is to always work on the depression. It is my experience that most people who have been diagnosed with depression are not depressed due to some genetic factor but, rather, because they are walking around thinking depressing thoughts. The natural treatment of depression is beyond the scope of this book; however, know that the majority of people can come out of depression by pursuing nondrug-related methods. A great resource is a book written many years ago by Dale Carnegie titled "*How to Stop Worrying and Start Living*."

Here is the bottom line: if you are depressed, you must be more aggressive at protecting your bones. All of the recommendations made thus far apply to you and should help to maintain your bones despite the depression. You may also want to become more aggressive at assessing your hormones and pursing such activities as yoga and meditation, which may help you enjoy better emotional balance.

Angry Neighbors Break Bones

I have a patient whom we shall call Mary (not her real name). Mary is 78 years old and takes great pride in the fact that she was using supplements over 30 years before it was "in style." Mary appears to be very healthy; she is extremely active and takes the blue ribbon for her homemade fudge and plants every year at the state fair. She eats well and stays active, and her checkups are typically very good.

One day, Mary awoke to find herself in excruciating back pain that became extremely debilitating. After a few days of trying to treat it herself, she finally decided to seek medical assistance. An X-ray of her back showed that Mary had broken a vertebra, and the DXA scan indicated that her bones were riddled with osteoporosis. After listening to Mary and getting a somewhat detailed health history, we could find no reason for her osteoporosis … until she started talking about her neighbor, who had terrorized her on a nearly daily basis for a number of years. As she spoke about the neighbor, I immediately realized that Mary's body had been in a constant state of stress, which had likely led to her bone eroding away. Can I be certain that this was the main cause of Mary's problem? No, admittedly I cannot, but in the absence of another cause I must acknowledge the 900 pound gorilla in the neighborhood.

Stress is like smoking: it can often negate the benefits of many other healthy efforts. If stress is a major issue for you, you must do something about it.

Chapter Summary:

There is no doubt that your mood impacts your health in many ways. Depression is considered a significant risk factor for osteoporosis and osteoporotic fracture. There are many reasons for this: 1. Behavioral factors that cause people to live indoors (less vitamin D), increased smoking, poorer diet, etc. 2. Medications commonly prescribed to depressed patients can increase the likelihood of osteoporosis and falls. 3. Stress hormones are produced in excess in depressed and anxious patients, which can erode the bones over time. 4. Depression and anxiety can inflame the body, which can lead to bone erosion. 5. Lower production of anabolic hormones in depressed patients can lead to less bone repair. 6. Depressed patients can often suffer from anxiety leading to prescriptions such as benzodiazepines which can lead to more falls. It would do your skeleton good to investigate non-drug approaches to treating depression such as counseling, exercise, yoga, and meditation. If, however, you need drug treatment then be diligent in every other aspect of your lifestyle described in the Strong Bones Forever book.

17

Supercharge Your Bone-Building Program

Throughout the program, we have covered the foundation for improving bone density and, more importantly, bone quality. In this chapter, I will cover other supplements that can significantly improve your results.

The supplements that we will discuss in this chapter include:

- Vitamin K
- Lycopene
- Melatonin
- Potassium
- Lycopene
- Green drinks

- CBD oil

I truly believe that every one of these supplements can provide significant benefits. I would even rank vitamin K and potassium as essential components of any serious bone-building program. I think you will see why once you read through this chapter.

Once the foundation program and these two essential nutrients have been implemented into your program; you can decide if you want to implement the other supplements as "icing on the cake."

Vitamin K – Super Vitamin for Building New Bone

Vitamin K is a fascinating nutrient, which scientists have rediscovered in recent years. Research indicates that vitamin K plays a very important role in balancing the body's biochemistry. These effects have been especially well documented with regard to blood coagulation (the ability of the blood to clot), vascular health, and bone mineralization.

Although vitamin K plays a vital role in many bodily processes, we are going to focus our discussion on its benefits to bone health. Vitamin K has some unique and extraordinary qualities. One interesting fact about vitamin K is that 75 percent of the vitamin K in our blood is actually produced made in our bodies. Keep in mind that our body cannot actually produce vitamins by definition, and vitamin K is no different. It is, in fact, the intestinal bacteria from in our body that produces the vitamin K. We will discuss the significance of this in greater detail later in the chapter.

Vitamins exist within two specific classes: water-soluble and fat-soluble vitamins. You may already know that vitamin K is considered a fat-soluble nutrient, but it is the only fat-soluble nutrient that does not store in the body. This means that you must either get vitamin K in the diet on a regular basis or the bacteria in your intestines must produce it each day in sufficient quantities to meet the body's needs. Unfortunately, for many people, the latter does not happen.

So Where Do We Get Vitamin K?

There are two types of vitamin K: vitamin K_1, and vitamin K_2. Vitamin K_1 is found in the diet within numerous foods, including green, leafy vegetables; green tea; and soybean oil. Vitamin K_2 is produced in the intestines by the intestinal bacteria. So why is vitamin K so deficient in our bodies?

We can answer that question first by looking at the diet of the standard American. As you already know, the Standard American Diet (SAD.) is very deficient in vegetables, which are the primary source of vitamin K_1 in the diet. Vitamin K balance is likely less of an issue for the minority of Americans who eat plenty of vegetables. In addition, vitamin K_1 is not the most active form of vitamin K, as it pertains to bone. Vitamin K_2, which is produced by the intestinal bacteria from vitamin K_1, is the active form of K and considered the most effective form for enhancing the growth and development of bones.

So much attention has been placed on minerals—such as calcium, magnesium, etc.—that we have left out the matrix of vital proteins that hold the minerals together like glue; without this biological glue, the minerals would have nothing to hold onto. This bone protein matrix is vital in the process of bone development and may, in fact, be the most important aspect. Vitamin K plays an important role in the production of a compound called GLA-containing proteins, which regulate many processes, including coagulation and bone mineralization. Most notably, vitamin K is utilized in the production of osteocalcin, the body's chief bone protein matrix. When vitamin K is deficient, osteocalcin cannot be produced; if this protein cannot be manufactured, then calcium, magnesium, and the other minerals will have nothing to hold onto once they reach the bone. Osteocalcin can be likened to the frame of a house, and minerals can be likened to the drywall that makes up the walls of the house. Without the frame, there is nothing to fasten the walls to, and the structure is weak.

Vitamin K deficiency has been shown to significantly increase the risk of osteoporosis and fractures. In fact, vitamin K status could possibly be a better predictor of bone fracture risk than bone density provided by the DXA scan. In recent years, studies have shown that vitamin K_1 and K_2 can improve bone formation in humans.

In one study conducted in Japan, researchers evaluated the blood levels of 24 women who had suffered osteoporotic fractures compared with 34 seniors who had not suffered osteoporotic fractures. Vitamin K_1 was virtually identical in both groups; however, vitamin K_2 levels were significantly lower in women who had suffered fractures and thus higher in people who seemed to have higher-quality bone.

More than a dozen studies on vitamin K in humans have proven vitamin K's ability to reverse or stabilize the disease. One study compared vitamin K with Fosamax and calcium alone. Both

Fosamax and vitamin K resulted in significantly lower fracture risk compared with calcium alone (*J Orthop Sci.* 2001;6:487–92.). I feel that the most important finding of this study is hidden behind the mechanism. Given the fact that vitamin K works through the production of osteocalcin, which is manufactured solely by the osteoblasts (bone builders), the likelihood is that vitamin K will result in higher-quality bone compared with Fosamax, even though the benefits to bone density are similar. Other studies have confirmed this benefit, some showing a synergistic effect with Fosamax and others showing synergistic effects with vitamin D. Vitamin K_2 has also been shown to benefit bone density in special populations, such as Parkinson patients, people with liver or kidney disease, and stroke victims. All of these populations are at significantly increased risk of osteoporosis and fracture.

Vitamin K is proving to be a very important anti-aging nutrient. Even though we have focused on bones in this discussion, vitamin K also has been shown to help regulate the clotting of the blood and to help remove calcium from the arteries. Although vitamin K is used in the clotting process, taking vitamin K in supplement form does not increase the risk of heart attack and stroke. In fact, through the normalization of the clotting process and the potential of vitamin K to remove calcium from the arteries, I feel that we will see significant decreases in both heart attack and stroke.

Vitamin K_2 comes in two forms: MK-4 and MK-7. MK-4 has been heavily studied and proven in high doses to be safe and effective at reversing osteoporosis. The recommended dose of vitamin K_2 (MK-4) is 15 mg three times daily. Less may be effective, but this is the dose that has been studied for reversing bone loss. There do not appear to be any side effects associated with this dosage. If you are on a blood thinner, such as warfarin (Coumadin), vitamin K is usually contraindicated. Talk to your doctor before adding vitamin K to your supplement program.

Vitamin K_1 and K_2 are both available. Although there is some research that suggests vitamin K_1 can convert into K_2 in the body's tissues, I feel that vitamin K_2 is more appropriate for those with osteoporosis. If you are looking to prevent osteoporosis, vitamin K_1 may be sufficient—but why risk it?

The MK-7 form of vitamin K_2 appears to be effective at lower doses and may prove to be more effective than the MK-4 form. I usually recommend a formula that delivers vitamin K_1 and both forms of vitamin K_2 in one formula. For recommendations, visit the website OsteoCoach.com/StrongBonesForever.

If you choose to get your vitamin K through the consumption of vegetables, then you must be especially vigilant at protecting the bacteria that reside in your gut. These bacteria will become the determining factor in how much benefit you will receive from the green, leafy vegetables. I would recommend supplementing with a probiotic supplement; specific recommendations

can be found at
OsteoCoach.com/StrongBonesForever.
One capsule daily can keep your body continuously colonized with healthy bacteria.

Protecting Your Body from Vitamin K2's Archenemy—K3

Having sufficient vitamin K_2 is only one piece of the "K Story." It turns out that an unhealthy lifestyle can inactivate healthy vitamin K_2 and result in a compound called K_3, formed from vitamin K_2 when we consume hydrogenated oils, trans fats, and acrylamides (compounds formed when starches are exposed to high heat). K_3 binds to receptors in the body and prevents vitamin K_2 from doing its very important job of regulating calcium levels. This just shows you how interconnected the body is. We must live healthy to be healthy. Even with proper supplementation, a poor lifestyle inactivates the best of efforts.

Lycopene – The Red Bone Builder

Researchers found an interesting correlation when they evaluated the dietary habits of a number of different cultures: they noticed that cultures that eat more tomatoes or tomato products suffered less fewer incidence of osteoporosis. It turns out that tomatoes are a wonderful source of a phytochemical called lycopene, which is the compound that gives tomatoes their red color. Lycopene is also found in strawberries, watermelons, and other red fruits and vegetables.

Leticia Rao, PhD, of the University of Toronto, found that lycopene was able to inhibit bone loss while simultaneously stimulating bone growth. We must question these findings, given the fact that the Heinz Corporation, which is a major distributor of tomato products, funded the research.

These results were also confirmed by other research that shows lycopene to be effective at inhibiting the growth of bone-breaking cells (osteoclasts). In addition, lycopene is a powerful antioxidant, and we know that oxidative free radicals have been correlated with increased risk of osteoporosis.

A study published in the journal *Osteoporosis International* examined 33 postmenopausal women and evaluated their risk of bone loss and how it correlated to their tomato intake. It was determined that the women with the highest tomato intake also had the least bone loss. The amount of tomato products consumed by the women with the lowest risk was just 2 tablespoons of tomato sauce or ketchup daily. You should note that when tomatoes are cooked, especially in an oil medium, the lycopene is liberated and the body is able to absorb this powerful compound with ease. This allows for smaller quantities to provide greater benefits.

So enjoy your tomato sauce, but go easy on the spaghetti and the pizza; the carbohydrates will most certainly negate the beneficial effects of the lycopene.

Lycopene is available in supplement form; but I do not recommend that you take products containing purified lycopene. Instead, look for fruit and vegetable concentrates that provide standardized levels of lycopene. Because fruits and vegetables are full of thousands of compounds, we must acknowledge that these other compounds could work with lycopene to benefit bone. You can find a number of supplements on the market that contain lycopene.

Melatonin – Sleep Your Way to Healthy Bones

There has been a lot of attention on sleep research and how healthy sleep patterns can significantly improve the quality of life as well as longevity. So much happens when we lie down to sleep at night. For instance, within the first hour after falling asleep, our body kicks out a big dose of growth hormone that stimulates repair and regeneration of many body tissues. Growth hormone is known as the hormone of youth, and some researchers even suggest that growth hormone injections may be a possible treatment for osteoporosis.

As fascinating and powerful as this hormone may be, it is not the topic of discussion in this section. Instead, I want to tell you about an inexpensive and safe nutritional supplement that is available at your local health-food store for pennies a day that may result in significant benefits to bones. Before we discuss this supplement, I feel it necessary to suggest that it is possible that this recommendation is a bit preliminary. I will give you arguments on both sides, give you my recommendation, and then send you on your way to make a decision.

There is a multitude of research on this supplement in test tubes, animals, and humans. It is considered to be very safe and effective as a tool to help you sleep. When it comes to the research on bone health, there is some rather interesting research in animals, test tubes, and, now, in humans.

Throughout this book, practically every scientific reference speaks of human studies, and, generally, I would not report on animal research. In this situation, however, there is other research, done on humans, to prove both benefits and safety.

The supplement I am referring to is melatonin, a hormone produced by the pineal gland when darkness falls. This hormone results in a smooth transition from the waking state of the day and the beginning process of preparing you for slumber. As we age, melatonin levels drop, and this decrease in circulating melatonin has been linked to many degenerative diseases.

Here is the jewel: in studies performed on rats, melatonin appears to stop bone loss and may even stimulate new bone growth. This benefit has been demonstrated in rats that have low estrogen levels and even in rats that were given steroids, such as methylprednisolone. As you know, steroids speed up bone loss, and melatonin appeared to protect them from steroid-induced bone loss.

Women who have lower amounts of nighttime melatonin in their bloodstream, such as shift-workers, are noted to suffer from lower bone density compared with women with normal blood melatonin levels.

Research into melatonin has discovered that it actually may stimulate the body to give birth to new bone-building cells and calms down overactive bone-breaking cells. In doing so, melatonin is not just slowing bone loss, but, rather, it is actually stimulating the sluggish bone-building cells to get to work.

Research in post-menopausal women with osteopenia (low bone density) found that melatonin supplementation resulted in a 2.2 percent increase in the femoral neck and a 3.6 percent increase in spinal bone density (*Journal of Pineal Research*. 59(2), 221–229).

Another study called the Melatonin-micronutrients Osteopenia Treatment Study (MOTS) looked at the effects of supplementing women with 5 mg of melatonin along with vitamin K_2, strontium, and vitamin D_3. After one year, the participants who were taking the melatonin and micronutrients enjoyed a 4.3 percent increase in the lumbar spine and a 2.2 percent increase in the femoral neck. These benefits were also backed up by the fact that blood testing confirmed the supplement group had a decrease in bone turnover (*Aging.* 2017 Jan; 9(1): 256–285).

Now, my recommendation: I feel that melatonin can be a useful tool in the prevention and treatment of bone loss, especially if you have trouble sleeping, regularly work the night shift, or are over age 50. For bone loss, I recommend 3 to 5 mg at night. If you find that you wake up groggy in the morning, then you may want to consider cutting the dose to between $1/2$ mg and $1\,1/2$ mg nightly.

As a final note, melatonin appears to play many important roles in the body besides its benefits with sleep. Melatonin appears to increase growth hormone secretion, may protect against breast cancer, and in some circles is used as an addition to treatment for women with breast cancer. It acts as a great antioxidant and plays a role in immune function.

Potassium – "I Shoulda Had a V8"

If you have read the chapter "The pH Factor," then you realize the importance of proper acid/base balance of the body. Calcium and magnesium play very important roles in bone health, but these two minerals reside deep in the bone. If the body dips into these stores, it means you have already burned through the bone's backup mineral reserves. These reserves are comprised of sodium and potassium, and are especially loosely bound to bone, which allows the body to grab and use them easily. This is what makes potassium such an important commodity to the body. If we provide the body with sufficient minerals to fill the reserves, then we can prevent it from dipping into the deeper calcium and magnesium reserves. This will protect the density of the bone.

Generally speaking, potassium in our bodies comes from a diet rich in fruits and vegetables. This means that if we get very few fruits and vegetables in the diet, then we will not meet the body's potassium needs. Several studies demonstrate the importance of a high fruit and vegetable diet in lowering the risk for osteoporosis. Other research correlates urine potassium levels with osteoporosis risk. Finally, the DASH Intervention Study demonstrates that eating 9 or 10 servings of fruits and vegetables per day can significantly decrease urinary calcium loss (*Am J Clin Nutr.* 2004;80(4):1019–23). Other research from the University of California shows that supplementing with potassium bicarbonate results in significant decreases in urinary calcium and phosphorous. In addition, the group that received the potassium also enjoyed less bone turnover, indicating a decreased loss of bone.

The recommended daily intake of potassium is 4,700 mg daily. You should try to get this dose through the foods you eat, which equates to approximately 8 cups of fruits and vegetables daily. If you find this difficult, then you can supplement with potassium in the dose of 400 mg three times daily. Potassium should be used cautiously, especially if you take medications for heart or blood pressure. If you are on these medications, please check with your doctor before you supplement with extra potassium. It is also important to note that the excess sodium intake in our diet further depletes the body of potassium.

Green Drink Powders

If you have already read "The pH Factor," then you already know of the importance of fruits and vegetables in maintaining blood pH. When the body is maintained at an acid pH, it must dip into the mineral bank account of the bones in order to correct the delicate balance within the blood and tissues.

Nature has placed within vegetables and fruits all the acid-neutralizing compounds needed to maintain the body's alkaline pH. These compounds include potassium, magnesium, sodium, calcium, and bicarbonate. In addition, there are many other phytochemicals, such as isoflavones, that work to inhibit inappropriate bone breakdown. The likelihood is that we have not even touched the surface of plant compounds that will prove to be beneficial to bone. We certainly have not been able to replicate the complex nutritional synergy that occurs within these colorful fruits and vegetables.

Research has shown that if we eat a lot of fruits and vegetables we can decrease calcium loss and inhibit bone breakdown. Unfortunately, many people find it difficult to meet these fruit and vegetable goals through diet alone. In addition, given all the environmental stresses that our bodies are under and the mineral depleted soils that the produce is grown in, it makes sense to use a green food powder on a daily basis to help meet the body's needs.

Green food powders are made from fruits and vegetables that are grown in mineral-rich, organic soils. They are then picked ripe, quickly frozen, and freeze-dried to be ground into a fine powder that can be reconstituted and taken as a fruit and vegetable supplement. This process helps to make available to the body the equivalent of two or three servings of fresh fruits and vegetables.

Is this the ideal way to take in fruits and vegetables? No, you can never beat eating the fruits and vegetables fresh, but the nutrition in these products clearly does help to balance maintain acid/base balance in the body and can be one more tool in the arsenal against osteoporosis.

Cannabidiol (CBD Oil) - Like Valium for Bone-Breakers

We have discussed the importance of bone-building cells and bone-breaking cells. The ultimate goal of a bone restoration program is not to simply stop bone-removing cells from chomping up bone; we also want to trigger the bone-building cells to get to work, while delivering the nutrients and building blocks needed to produce healthy bone.

During the course of this book, I have beaten up on osteoporosis drugs because of the way they work by poisoning bone-breaking cells to the point where they commit cell-suicide through a process that scientists call apoptosis. Sadly, this process of permanent cell-death leads to poor-quality bone over time, due to the fact that bone-breaking cells and bone-building cells work together to remove old bone and to build new, healthy bone. Without one, the other does not work effectively. What if there was a way to turn the volume down on the bone-removing cells without killing them off? What if we could simply normalize and optimize bone-removing cells so that the bone builders could simply catch up? What if we could do this with a safe and readily available supplement that can be bought at practically any health-food store in the United States?

Researchers uncovered a receptor, called the GPR55 receptor, which can be found on osteoclast cells, that when activated increases the activity and speed of bone breakdown. Once discovered, scientists then tested and confirmed that if they block the receptor, the bone-breaking cells take a nap and slow down significantly.

Soon it was discovered that a natural compound called CBD oil could bind to and block the GRP55 receptor, thus slowing the osteoclasts in laboratory animals. The result was that experimental fractures in lab animals healed much faster than within the group given a placebo (*Proceedings of the National Academy of Sciences,* September 2009). This is fascinating and encouraging data because osteoporosis drugs, which take a sledgehammer to the bone breakers, have been shown to *slow* bone healing after fractures.

A more recent study, once again involving rodents, found that CBD oil prevented bone loss in rats with a spinal cord injury, with the inner bone (trabecular bone) showing enhanced bone volume in CBD-treated rats (*European Journal of Pharmacology,* August 2017).

Admittedly, the research on CBD oil is in its infancy, especially concerning bone loss. That being said, mechanistically CBD oil appears to be a safe and potentially effective tool in the fight against bone loss. I have used CBD oil very successfully in my practice to help with pain, inflammation, anxiety, PTSD, and memory loss. We can now add osteoporosis to the list of potential benefits, something I hope will be confirmed in human trials soon.

If you would like to try CBD oil for osteoporosis, I recommend killing two birds with one stone and using a formula that combines CBD oil with melatonin. If you suffer from pain, inflammation, anxiety, PTSD, or memory loss, you may want to consider taking CBD oil up to three times daily in doses between 5 to 50 mg three times daily. It has been a godsend for many of my patients and may provide other benefits advantages besides potential benefit to bone. There are many formulas on the market and recommendations change with time, so I will not recommend a specific brand here. For an impartial recommendation, visit OsteoCoach.com/StrongBonesForever.

Chapter Summary:

Vitamin K is a very important nutrient for building healthy bones. Without vitamin K the body cannot build the scaffolding needed to lay down minerals and thus harden the bones. Vitamin K_2 is considered the most important form of vitamin K for bones. Aside from vitamin K, other supplements may also improve bone resilience such as melatonin, lycopene, green drink powders, and CBD oil.

18

The OsteoCoach Approach - Build Your Bone Resilience Action Plan

Now that you have a comprehensive understanding of the science behind how to build bone, we need to combine those tactics into a strategy that you can implement into your life. In this chapter, we will focus in on how to use this knowledge and assemble these tactics into a complete strategy for building resilient bones.

Step 1: Build Your Bone-Building Supplement Program

As we discussed, we need to make sure that your bones have sufficient building blocks so that when we trigger the bone-building cells, they will have the necessary materials to build a healthy bone matrix that will be fracture resistant. Due to the fact that my supplement recommendations change as new science comes to light and new products come to market, I will not make specific recommendations of brands and products here. If you would like my latest product recommendations, they are available for free as a *Strong Bones Forever* bonus at www.OsteoCoach.com/StrongBonesForever. In this section, I will focus on recommendations of nutrients and doses.

Nutrient Recommendation #1: Bone Mineral Formula

As you know, I do not recommend a "calcium" supplement because the bones require more than calcium to grow stronger. Instead, we recommend a comprehensive "bone mineral formula." A good bone mineral formula will provide the following nutrients in the minimal doses described:

1. Calcium (as MCHA, citrate, malate, lactate, chelate, etc.): 400 to 800 mg per day. If you follow the recommendations in the diet chapter of this book, you will be getting 600 to 800 mg of calcium from food, so you will need only an extra 400 to 800 mg to meet your body's needs for the day. Avoid calcium carbonate, but almost any other form will suffice. See chapter 9, The Calcium Controversy, for more specific recommendations.

2. Magnesium (as citrate, malate, glycinate, chelate, aspartate, orotate, etc.): 400 to 800 mg per day. Magnesium is very important for healthy bones and may in fact be more important than calcium due to the fact that it is more commonly deficient in most people's diets. We aim for a calcium/magnesium ratio of

1:1 (1 mg of magnesium per 1 mg of calcium), but anywhere between 1:1 and 2:1 should be fine.
3. Boron (the preferred form is fructoborate, but other forms such as citrate, are fine, too): 3 to 6 mg per day
4. Silica: 5 to 25 mg per day
5. Zinc (as citrate, picolinate, monomethionine, etc.): 5 to 25 mg per day
6. Copper (citrate is common; most forms are fine): 0.5 to 1.5 mg per day
7. Manganese (citrate is common; most forms are fine): 5 to 10 mg per day
8. Strontium (citrate is common; most forms are fine): 0.5 to 6 mg per day. I do not recommend dosing higher than 10 mg per day.

Nutrient Recommendation #2: Vitamin D3 (Cholecalciferol)

Our goal is to supplement with sufficient vitamin D_3 to bring our blood levels up to the optimal range of 50 to 70 ng/ml. Most adults can achieve this with 2,000 to

5,000 IU per day. If you do not have a blood test to guide your dosage, I recommend starting with 4,000 IU per day. If you have had a recent blood test, a good guideline to follow is 1,000 IU per 10 point increase needed. For example, if your blood test shows a blood level of 20 ng/ml and you want to increase your vitamin D to 50 ng/ml, then you will need to supplement with a minimum of 3,000 IU daily. These are just guidelines and follow-up blood tests will determine if you are taking sufficient quantities of vitamin D_3. Note: Most doctors prescribe vitamin D_2 (ergocalciferol), but this is an inferior form so you may want to speak to your doctor about switching to daily vitamin D_3. Vitamin D_3 is quite safe, and most people can safely use up to 5,000 IU daily without worry of toxicity, even if you do not have blood tests. If you are thin, you may need less; if you are heavy, you may need 5,000 to 10,000 IU to reach optimal blood levels.

Nutrient Recommendation #3: Vitamin K2

Vitamin D helps to carry minerals into the bloodstream, and vitamin K helps to direct those minerals into the bones. Vitamin K is also very important in keeping calcium out of the arteries. Dosages will vary depending on the form of vitamin K that you are taking. Although all three forms of vitamin K (K_1, MK-4, and MK-7) are important to health, the two forms of vitamin K_2 (MK-4 and MK-7) are most beneficial to bone. For simplicity, I recommend between 150 to 180 mcg of MK-7 per day. That being said, in my practice, I use a formula that combines the three forms of vitamin K together. See the free resources at www.OsteoCoach.com/StrongBonesForever for my latest recommendations.

Nutrient Recommendation #4: Collagen Peptide Powder

Besides vitamins and minerals, the other building block of bone is protein. Collagen is a form of protein used in both bones and joints, acting as scaffolding for minerals. Collagen peptides help to improve the ability of bone builders to lie down and harden new bone. As a side note, people who supplement with collagen peptides report improve joint health and healthier, younger-looking skin. Recommended dose: 20 grams twice daily.

Step 2: Begin a Walking Program and Aim for 10,000 Steps per Day

In the previous chapters, I reported on the negative effects of microgravity caused by near-constant sitting and lying down. The more you walk, the more your bone cells will work. Although walking is likely more beneficial for maintaining or slowing bone loss, it is still important for health. To add extra stimulus to the bones, consider using a weighted vest when walking. Also consider using walking poles for added stability to decrease the risk of falls.

Step 3: Expose Your Body to Osteogenic Stimulation

Osteogenic stimulation involves loading the body with sufficient stimulus to trigger the bone remodeling process for stronger and denser bone. You achieve this through resistance training and most notably when you expose your bones to loads that are four times your bodyweight. The best technology for achieving osteogenic loads to the bone is called BioDensity, and you can find a center near you by visiting their website Biodensity.com. If you are in the Baltimore area, visit the OsteoCoach Center for Strong Bones in Owings Mills. If you do not have access to a BioDensity machine near you, then I recommend starting a resistance training program. Start with lighter weights that allow you to perform 12 to 15 repetitions; as you get stronger, increase the weight to a load that allows you to perform only 6 to 8 repetitions. Resistance training is vital for building a healthy skeleton and body. Do not skip this step as it will mean the difference between slowing or maintaining your current bone density as well as dramatically increasing your bone density over time.

Running and sprinting is another way to expose your body to an osteogenic load; however, most people with osteopenia and osteoporosis cannot safely implement such a program. Alternatively, you may want to look into a vibration plate as discussed in the chapter 13, Exercising Your Right to Strong Bones, I should note that osteogenic loading is likely the most important step in your bone-building program. Even with a mediocre diet and supplementation, osteogenic loading has demonstrated dramatic improvements in bone strength.

Step 4: Limit the Use of Drugs That May Deplete Your Bones

The most common drugs that can do a number on your bone strength and quality are antacid medications and steroids. Revisit chapter 12, Inflammation and Medications – Enemies of the Skeleton, for more information on inflammation and drugs and how they impact your skeleton.

Step 5: Review the Chapter on the Perfect 10-Point Diet

In the book, I outlined 10 ways to improve your diet for healthy bones. Review chapter 14, The Perfect Bone-Building Diet and implement as many of the recommendations as possible. Diet is extremely important to building healthy bones and, like resistance exercise, should not be ignored. You can change your bones by changing your diet. Follow these recommendations: 1. Eat 3 times more vegetables, nuts, and seeds than meat or refined carbohydrates 2. Stop drinking soda 3. Limit sugar and refined carbohydrates 4. Limit sodium 5. Consume healthy omega-3 fats from nuts, seeds, and fish 6. Drink 60-80 ounces of water daily 7. Eat lean protein 8. Limit dairy 9. Limit coffee 10. Limit alcohol.

This is a big book to summarize in just five simple steps, my hope is that these steps will provide you with the 20% that delivers 80% of the benefits. If you do just these five steps, you will build strong bones forever! My hope is that you have learned that a low bone density isn't a guarantee that you will fracture a bone. You can change your lifestyle, diet, exercise plan, and supplement program to build a stronger, healthier, and resilient skeleton. Shifting your lifestyle in this way can increase your chances of living a life on your terms, without need to depend on anyone. Unlike the drugs prescribed for osteoporosis, this program has only positive side effects. As you follow the instructions in this program you will enjoy more energy, more physical strength, healthier joints, more vitality, a healthier mood, and the wellbeing of someone twenty years younger.

19

In Case of Hip-Fracture, Break Glass - A Guide to Surviving a Hip Fracture

Recently, I received an email from the family of a woman I had briefly met a couple of years ago at a conference. I was unaware that she suffered from osteoporosis but learned that she had fallen and fractured her hip. According to the email, she made it through the surgery just fine, but while in the hospital, she developed a clot in the leg; a piece of that clot broke off and traveled to the lung, called a pulmonary embolism. The pulmonary embolism was very serious, and she died shortly thereafter. Although I did not know her well, nor had I ever discussed osteoporosis with her, I was taken aback by her unfortunate story. It never had occurred to me to write about how to survive a hip fracture because my life is dedicated to the prevention of disease and the promotion of vitality and health. As I thought about it, I realized that, although my life is dedicated to improving bone strength and preventing fractures, people may not get this information in time.

Improving the strength of bones takes time. because Because many people who order this book are further along in the progress of the disease, I feel it necessary to write this report. Some of you may have recently been diagnosed with mild bone loss, while others may have already lost greater than 50 percent of bone mass. Still, others have family members with osteoporosis and are looking for alternatives for their loved ones. Although I like to fantasize that everybody who orders this book gets it in their hands early in the course of their condition, I must admit that this will simply not be the case. It is my prayer that none of you go on to develop a hip fracture, but should disaster strike, I want to give you the information you need to make informed decisions and the tools that you need to stack the cards in your favor. Thus I present to you "In Case of Hip Fracture, Break Glass—A Guide to Surviving a Hip Fracture."

Scope of the Problem

Every year, it is estimated that 300,000 unlucky souls suffer hip fractures. Although there are also 700,000 spinal fractures, 250,000 wrist fractures, and 300,000 fractures of other bones, none of them are as devastating as the dreaded hip fracture, which you will learn, is all too often deadly.

After a hip fracture, it is estimated that one in three people will not make it to see their next birthday. Just writing that sentence sends shivers down my spine. Keeping that in mind, there are two questions to consider as they relate to hip fractures:

1. What determines who lives and who dies?
2. What can we do to increase your chances of surviving a hip fracture and the impending surgery?

First, let us discuss the factors that place you at risk of succumbing to a hip fracture. By the way, if some of these factors describe you, do not worry; I will help you to formulate a plan that will help stack the cards in your favor.

In a large-scale study, scientists evaluated 11 disease factors, called comorbidities, that could potentially worsen your chances of survival. I have designed the questionnaire below to help you figure out which apply to you.

- Do you have heart disease? Answer "yes" if you have had a heart attack or heart arrhythmia, or if your doctor has told you that you are at risk of having a heart attack.
- Have you ever had a stroke?
- Do you suffer from respiratory diseases, such as COPD, poorly controlled asthma, emphysema, or pulmonary fibrosis?

- Do you have diabetes?
- Do you suffer from rheumatoid arthritis?
- Do you suffer from Parkinson's disease?
- Do you have cancer?
- Do you suffer from Paget's disease?
- Are you currently a smoker?
- Do you currently take any steroids, such as prednisone?

Count Your Yeses: _____

Not unexpectedly, the more questions for which you answered yes, the higher the chances that you will end up with complications after a hip fracture. If you answered no to all questions, then congratulations, you have the lowest risk of complications. The paragraphs that follow will compare your results with people who answered no to all questions. Once again, this is not meant to scare you, it simply gives us a "you are here" perspective, which we can use to formulate a plan.

To summarize, the more disease factors that you have (yes answers to the above questions), the higher your risk of developing complications after surgery and possibly succumbing to one of those complications. In a nutshell, the healthier you are when you are admitted, the better you will do while in the hospital. I admit that is not groundbreaking news. With that said, I feel that we tend to forget the importance of overall health, and sometimes need to be reminded of the obvious in order to begin again to build health and vitality, before catastrophe strikes. If you are reading this report preemptively, having never suffered a fracture, then take that message to heart and do everything that you can to strengthen your muscles and to remain well nourished and generally healthy. Of course, follow the *Strong Bones Forever* program to begin the process of strengthening bones and body so that you never have to refer to this report ever again.

The Sicker You Are, the Higher Your Risk

The more comorbidities you have, the higher the risk for complications and/or death. If you answered yes to one of the questions, your risk of death is 30 percent higher than if you answered no to all questions. If you answered yes to two of the questions, your risk is 70 percent higher. If you answered "yes" to three or more of the questions, your risk goes up 140 percent. As you can see, the more illnesses you have, the higher your risk. No news here. Perhaps you are not as interested in the exact number; perhaps you are more interested in what this means to the plan.

To put it simply, the more dismal the potential outcome, the more you have to fight to avoid becoming a statistic. This will often mean being more assertive and active in the process of developing your health plan. You simply cannot rely on the hospital to look out for your well-being, as their best efforts place you at a 1-in-3 risks of succumbing to the disaster within the next year. To stack the cards in your favor, you will have to take a more active role in formulating a plan to "Survive and

Thrive." We will get to that in a moment
…

After the Fracture

After the hip fracture event, the research suggests that you will fare better if you get into surgery within 24 hours of the accident. Do not let doctors delay due to limited resources (such as operating room space). Remember, the squeaky wheel gets the grease. If you make it clear to them that you understand that surgical intervention within 24 hours of fracture results in improved outcomes, this may place you at the top of their list of priorities for fear of malpractice retaliation. Simply give them stern instructions to go to surgery as soon as possible, unless there are extenuating circumstances that may increase the risk of complications during surgery (significant heart failure may be such an issue). If they feel that surgery may be too risky, I would defer to their judgment. Become assertive only when the reason they give has more to do with the availability of doctor's time and/or an operating room availability. Be polite but assertive; you want your doctors to *want* you to get better, and the truth of the matter is, it helps if they like you.

The Biggest Risks

Of all the health issues that place you at greatest risk for having complications, the following issues are most important:

1. Kidney disease
2. Respiratory problems
3. Cancer (current)
4. Current use of steroids (such as prednisone)
5. Parkinson's disease

There are other factors that impact the risk of complications, but these are the most likely factors to pose a problem. Although not sufficiently studied in the research literature, I would also include unstable heart failure (congestive heart failure). We will discuss this when we get to post-surgical complications. If you suffer from any of the above-mentioned health problems when you are/were admitted to the hospital after a hip fracture, then you are automatically considered high risk.

Complications After Surgery

It is well documented that heart failure and/or chest infections are considered the most dangerous post-surgical complications. We know that kidney disease, respiratory problems, and steroid use predispose you to either heart failure and/or chest infection, which may be why they are such important risk factors for poor outcomes after surgery. It is also vital to note that the more complications you have after surgery, the higher the likelihood of a bad outcome. In fact, having just one complication increases your risk of dying within the next 30 days by 5.6 times; if you have two complications after surgery, your risk of dying within 30 days goes up by 13 times.

Understanding Heart Failure

Heart failure occurs when the heart is unable to meet the demands of the body. This occurs for a number of reasons:

1. The heart muscle gets weak and cannot move enough blood through the circulatory system to feed the organs.
2. The heart muscle is normal, but the electrical activity of the heart has gone haywire. An example of this is atrial fibrillation. Heart arrhythmias can decrease the amount of blood that is being pumped through the circulatory system.
3. Valve problems can decrease the cardiac output by allowing blood to flow back into the chamber in between heartbeats. In a normal heart, the valve prevents regurgitation of blood once it gets pressed into circulation. Diseased valves can allow blood to "fall" back into the heart. This is the proverbial "two steps forward and one step back."

4. High blood pressure can increase the demand on the heart. When blood pressure is excessively high, the heart must work harder to move the volume of blood needed to keep the organs working. Sometimes, the heart just is not strong enough to push blood against such high pressure.
5. Some medications can weaken the heart and decrease output. There are too many medications with this side effect to list here, but the most common drugs are statin medications, beta-blockers, and other heart medications.

Heart failure is a major concern after surgery. Although only 13 percent of hip fracture patients develop heart failure, this complication is responsible for 73 percent of deaths within the first 30 days post-surgery. That makes heart failure your number one foe. After surgery it is important that you report excess fluid in the legs and/or shortness of breath as these may be signs of heart failure.

Kidney disease can stack the cards against you in a number of ways:

1. Kidney failure can cause fluid retention, which increases blood pressure.
2. Kidney failure can lead to anemia, which will require the heart to move more blood to properly oxygenate the tissues.
3. Kidney failure may negatively impact mineral balance within the body.
4. Kidney failure can negatively impact the metabolism of vitamin D needed for bone healing.

Prednisone and other corticosteroids:

1. Cause sodium and fluid retention, which increases blood pressure.
2. Decrease the proper healing of tissues.
3. Decrease immune response to infection.

4. Prevent the proper repair of bone.
5. Increase mineral loss, which can limit the building blocks available for repairing the bone after surgery.

Parkinson's Disease (PD)

1. PD increases the likelihood of falls by 300 percent.
2. Patients with PD have limited ability to move around, which may negatively impact physical therapy and recovery.
3. PD patients are already at risk of low bone density and, therefore, increased fracture risk.

Cancer

1. Cancer increases the risk of bone metastases, which can lead to bone fractures.
2. Cancer treatment can promote bone loss.
3. Cancer treatment can result in problems with balance.

4. Treatment for cancer may inhibit immune function and increase the chance of infection.
5. Physical resources within the body may be allocated toward the repair of other tissues rather than bone.

How Do We Use This Information?

I am going to speak to this question on two fronts: First, I will speak to steps you can take within the hospital to prevent postsurgical complications; then I will speak to nutritional or complementary interventions that may help to improve outcomes after surgery.

Conventional Thinking on Preventing Complications

Unfortunately, there is little research around interventions for preventing complications after hip surgery. Because research is limited, I will recommend certain steps that may help you to uncover hidden factors that may increase your risk of complication. This will allow your doctors to take preemptive steps to manage these complications. In other words, your chances improve if someone is on guard against signs and symptoms of complications.

Here is how to utilize hospital resources to protect you from complications:

1. Request that specialists do a pre- and postsurgery evaluation in order to assess the risk of cardiac and respiratory complications. With heart failure accounting for the biggest risk of complication, the cardiology department of the hospital should assess the cardiac output, blood pressure, electrolytes, and medications for factors that may place you (or your loved one) at risk.
2. If you suffer from pulmonary problems, request that a pulmonary specialist assess you for the presence of and risk of respiratory infection. Ask if there is any

procedure that they can implement that will prevent such infections after surgery.

3. If you suffer from heartburn or reflux, be careful to do everything in your power to prevent such reflux episodes, as this can increase your risk of infection. This occurs when food material and stomach juices reflux up into the esophagus and fall back into the windpipe. Most doctors will simply prescribe antacid medications; although this may decrease the heartburn symptoms, it does nothing to prevent reflux. If you suffer from bad reflux, bring this up with your physician and inquire about preventative antibiotics. Request smaller, more frequent meals. Also, request that the head remain elevated if possible, as this will decrease the chances that food will reflux into the lungs.

4. If you suffer from kidney problems, request evaluations from kidney and cardiac specialists. The goal here is to make sure that all electrolyte imbalances (potassium, sodium,

magnesium) are aggressively treated prior to surgery. Also, make sure that the blood pressure is neither too strong nor too weak to maintain healthy circulation.

5. If you take steroids, such as prednisone, inform the surgeon and attending physician so that they can keep a close eye out for respiratory infection.

6. Make sure that the doctors keep a close eye on monitor for postoperative oxygen saturation (how much oxygen is dissolved in your blood). Blood oxygen is important in order to assure proper healing after surgery. In addition, a decrease in oxygen saturation could indicate heart failure or infection.

7. Blood clots are an important risk factor after leg and hip surgeries. Inquire about the hospital's plan and procedure for making sure that clots do not develop. Usually, this could involve procedures for keeping the limbs moving at regular intervals, medications to prevent clots, hydration plans, therapy, massage,

etc. The bottom line is, there should be a plan for preventing blood clots. You may want to familiarize yourself with signs and symptoms of blood clots, such as pain or hotness in the lower leg (beneath the knee) and sudden onset of breathing difficulties. After surgery, you will have limited mobility and may not realize that a clot has formed; request that the nurses check you regularly for leg clots. The point is, keep an eye out for clots, but more importantly, find out how the hospital intends to prevent the clot from forming in the first place. Sudden pain in the chest or shortness of breath can indicate a clot in the lungs. Report any unusual sensations in the chest to the attending nurse and doctor.

8. If your bones do not seem to be healing after surgery, ask the doctor to get you to a hyperbaric oxygen chamber. After a fracture, bones may not fuse properly; this could be attributed to poor circulation to the affected bone. Some research has found that such situations can be

helped by hyperbaric oxygen treatment. This treatment involves sitting or lying in a chamber that delivers oxygen to the body under high pressure. This forces more oxygen into the blood, which stimulates healing.

Complementary Approach to Improving Outcomes

In addition to the eight points listed above, I would like to spend some time discussing some other factors that may improve your chances of coming out of surgery with fewer complications.

The Common Sense Advice You Must Hear Again!

You no doubt have heard the old cliché "an ounce of prevention is worth a pound of cure." I debated whether to add this section for fear that you may view it as common sense or an insult to your intelligence. However, in my experience, people must be reminded of this important factor in order for them to eventually act on it. I feel that the biggest reason people do not want to hear about prevention is that they do not see what an enormous impact a proper preventive program can have on their health and lives. They lie in their hospital beds, recuperating from hip surgery, saying to themselves, *How could I be so stupid? Why did I try to pick up that box when I know I have poor balance?* or *Why did I not turn the light on when I got up in the middle of the night to go to the bathroom?* Do not be that person. If, however, you are already "that person," then learn from it and vow to never let it happen again. Below are my recommendations for preventing fractures and improving the likelihood of a healthy recovery in the unfortunate circumstance of a hip fracture:

1. The Instant Cure for Hip Fractures

There is only one instant cure for hip fractures: <u>never have one</u>. Many of the recommendations that we make in this program can have a delayed benefit; a change made today may not reap fruit for many months. One recommendation, however, can have instantaneous benefit: we are beginning to hear a lot about what are called low-force or low-impact fractures; these are basically fractures that occur for no apparent reason, such as walking or standing in a subway train. These fractures are odd and newsworthy, and we should pay attention to them. However, we must not lose sight of the fact that the great majority of osteoporotic fractures occur only after a significant fall or blunt force. If we could significantly decrease the likelihood of falling, we can significantly as well as instantaneously decrease the likelihood that you will end up lying in a hospital bed with this manual in hand. This will also allow us the time needed to promote new, strong, pliable bone to develop.

2. Strengthen your muscles

Improving the strength of your muscles should be a priority in your fracture-prevention program. Aside from the benefits to bone structure and strength, muscle also acts as a shock absorber when the body is struck with blunt force. The thicker your muscle, the less force will be distributed to the bones. Imagine that I had you stand in front of me, and I informed you that I was going to punch you in the gut. Before I do that, however, I offer you two options for protective gear: a 1-inch-thick pillow or a 1-inch-thick piece of hard rubber. Which would you choose? If you picked the pillow, well, you better prepare yourself to have the wind knocked out of you. You may have been lulled by the softness of the pillow, but soft materials allow too much force to make it through. Harder materials distribute the force to a wider surface area, which results in less force being distributed to a single point.

A good example of this is the magician's trick in which he lies on a bed of nails. Because there are so many nails distributed across the whole area of his body, the nails never puncture the skin.

What do you think would happen if he tried to lie on a single nail? Ouch! The entire force of the body, 200 or so pounds, would be distributed to one point: the sharp point of the nail. How does this apply to our discussion? The muscle acts as hard rubber. The more toned the muscle and the thicker the pad of muscle, the more force your body will be able to absorb without developing a fracture.

Aside from protecting the body from blunt force and strengthening bone, muscle also acts as a depot for protein building blocks. During times of illness, such as after a fracture or surgery, your body can turn to the protein in muscle to fuel itself. Recent research suggests that the more muscle you have on your body, the lower your risk of developing an infection. This means more muscle results in better immune function.

The best way to improve muscle tone and size is through weight lifting and resistance training. I recommend that you seek out guidance when beginning a weight-training program so that you can learn how to train safely and effectively.

3. Train Your Muscles

In addition to building bigger and denser muscle mass, training your muscles in certain ways can promote better gait, balance, and ability to recover from situations in which you begin to fall. Training muscles for improved balance is slightly different than training for improved strength, tone, and thickness. It is true that any resistance-training program will likely improve balance, but some kinds of training, known as functional training, can help to improve the connection between your brain and muscles.

In a nutshell, nerves exit the spinal cord and reach out to the muscles to allow the brain to connect to and control muscle contractions. Some of these contractions are controlled by your conscious mind while others, such as balance, are controlled by your subconscious mind. By training in a functional manner, you will work to improve control of the small movements of the muscles needed for proper balance. At the end of the nerve, small fingers protrude to activate the muscle. The more of these little "nerve-fingers" that you have, the better able your brain will be to monitor and to keep your body in balance. Resistance exercise, especially functional training, helps to promote the sprouting of more nerve-fingers to better control micromovements of the muscles that you need to stay in balance. Balance training can be performed at home as well. The good news is that nerves respond quickly to any resistance training. It is not uncommon for people to see improved balance and strength within a matter of two or three weeks after starting a program. This benefit occurs because of improved nerve connection to the muscle.

Another way to improve balance is through the use of low-intensity vibration training, discussed in chapter 13, Exercise Your Right To Strong Bones. If financially feasible, I highly recommend purchasing a Marodyne LIV and using it for 10 minutes daily to improve balance and bone health. You can order the Marodyne LIV by visiting OsteoCoach.com.

4. Decrease or Eliminate Unnecessary Medications

Due to the constantly changing nature of medicine, the medical industry has become very specialized. In fact, it is not uncommon for a patient to have a general practitioner, endocrinologist, cardiologist, gynecologist, gastroenterologist, orthopedist, and neurologist. Each of these doctors works within their niche to treat particular diseases and health challenges. Unfortunately, there is little cross talk between all these various specialists, and the results can be catastrophic. For example, if you go to a cardiologist's office, she may treat your blood pressure problem without considering the possibility that a medication may lower blood pressure too far, resulting in dizziness and a fall that could land you in the hospital with a hip fracture. One of the most common causes of falls in seniors is from the use of blood pressure medications, antidepressants, anxiety medications, and/or sleep medication that were prescribed by general practitioners or neurologists without considering the possible ramifications of these prescriptions for fracture risk.

These are just some examples of an infinite list of possibilities. There are healthcare practitioners who specialize in helping seniors safely decrease unnecessary or unproven drug therapies. They are especially adept at analyzing the benefit/risk ratio of drug treatment in order to promote the best outcomes in patients. If you take numerous medications, I would seek out a specialist in the area of geriatric medicine or "poly-pharmacy" and instruct them to strip your program down to the bare minimum.

5. Follow The Strong Bones Forever Program

Early in the *Strong Bones Forever* program, I mentioned that what fixes your bones also seems to fix your body. By putting the recommendations of this program into action, you will build a level of health that will astound you and your doctor. Aside from improving bone density, decreasing fracture risk, and feeling more confident on your feet, you will also be improving your body's ability to bounce back from injury, illness, and unexpected fractures.

A study published September 9, 2010, in the *Journal of the American Geriatrics Society* found that there are different risk factors for falls that occur indoors versus falls that occur outdoors. According to the study, approximately one-half of falls occur indoors and one-half occur outdoors. The people who fell indoors had a tendency to be less active, had more physical disabilities, had poorer cognitive function, and took more medications than those who fell outdoors. Those patients who fell outdoors were more likely to be male, seemed to have healthier lifestyles, and trended toward having more education. Up to this point, the interventions to prevent falls have centered on strengthening and gait activities, as well as on obstacle-management within the home. According to the researchers of this study, it now appears that such interventions will impact only one-half of the falls that occur. We now must develop a set of interventions for prevention of outdoor falls that are different from those designed to prevent indoor falls. My intention is to alert you to this finding so that you will be more cognizant of the potential to fall and fracture a bone while out and about. Let me be clear, it is not my intention to turn you into a recluse. I feel that you should not live in fear of falls; rather, you should educate yourself and do everything in your power to keep your eyes open for situations and obstacles that may place you at risk. Some of these obstacles include:

- Sidewalks
- Curbs (especially unpainted curbs)
- Uneven surfaces
- Outdoor debris

Taking Steps to Improve Outcomes After Hip Fracture

Admittedly, many of the recommendations that I will make in this part of the report are based on years of experience and educated hypotheses. In the absence of studies that have specifically evaluated these recommendations against risk of complications after hip fracture, I must extrapolate from other research and make an educated guess as to how it could benefit you during that trying time. These would be interventions that I would make for myself or with my own family if I were faced with a hip fracture situation. Typically, I do not like to write about educated guesses, however, I am comforted by three facts:

1. These interventions will not harm; they will only provide benefits.
2. Although there is no specific research with these products as they relate to hip fracture, there is plenty of published literature that suggests safety and efficacy in related situations.
3. There is a solid theoretical reason to believe that they would benefit someone who is recuperating from a hip fracture.

Let us start with a common denominator among people who suffer with heart failure, kidney dysfunction, heart valve problems, immune problems, cancer, and Parkinson's disease. Yes, there is a common denominator that could predispose a person to any and all of these conditions. There is also plenty of research that suggests that correcting this common deficiency can actually slow or even reverse these conditions.

Many years ago, scientists discovered a compound within the human body that seemed to play a major role in the production of energy within the cells. In fact, when they looked at the various tissues and cells of the body, they discovered this compound in all of them. The scientists called this compound ubiquinone because it was so ubiquitous in the body. You may know it as coenzyme Q10 (CoQ10).

CoQ10 is found across the United States as a nutritional supplement and available without a prescription. In fact, coenzyme Q10 is so effective it is used as a prescription treatment in Japan for heart failure.

Research in the States and abroad has discovered that when the body's CoQ10 levels drops by 25 percent the cells can become dysfunctional. This dysfunction can culminate in disease, which include:

1. Heart failure
2. Kidney failure
3. Brain disease
4. Fatigue
5. Immune dysfunction
6. Cancer
7. Heart disease

When the CoQ10 levels drops to 25 percent or less, meaning dropped by 75 percent of normal level, you basically cannot produce sufficient cellular energy to survive and thus you die. That just goes to show you how important CoQ10 is to the body. It is important to note that the tissues that have to work the hardest require the most energy, and thus are the ones that are most susceptible to disease caused by CoQ10 deficiency. These include the brain, heart, kidney, liver, immune system, and muscles.

What Causes CoQ10 Deficiency?

Coenzyme Q10 is not a vitamin because the body has the capacity to produce its own CoQ10. Coenzyme Q10 deficiency can occur for many reasons. However, the two most common are:

1. Age: After age 50, Coenzyme Q10 deficiency can become an issue.
2. Medications: There are many prescription drugs that interfere with the body's ability to produce CoQ10. The most common drugs are statins (such as Lipitor®, Crestor®, Zocor®) and other heart medications (such as beta-blockers). I would recommend that you look into all of your medications to see if they might promote a deficiency of CoQ10.

How Should I Use CoQ10?

There are two forms of CoQ10 on the market: ubiquinol and ubiquinone. Ubiquinol is the superior form of coenzyme Q10 because it is pre-activated, better absorbed, and stays in the bloodstream longer than ubiquinone. I recommend most people use the ubiquinol form of CoQ10.

If you are generally healthy and are looking to keep your CoQ10 levels in the normal, healthy range, I recommend 100 mg per day. If you have any of the previously mentioned diseases or medications, you may need to take 200 to 300 mg per day, in divided doses. If you have had a hip fracture and have had surgery and/or are preparing for surgery, I would recommend 300 to 400 mg be taken prior to and/or after surgery. CoQ10 has been studied in people who were undergoing open-heart surgery. Not only was the CoQ10 safe for use with such a surgery, but also the people who took the CoQ10 enjoyed better outcomes. During open-heart surgery, the surgeons have to stop the heart from beating until the work is done. Surgeons have found that the hearts of patients who were pretreated with CoQ10 started back up much more easily than the placebo group. In addition, they noted less damage to the heart after surgery. Although presurgical CoQ10 may be quite beneficial, it is better for you to have been taking CoQ10 prior to admission. This would make CoQ10 a good product to add to your overall health and wellness regimen.

Two Nutrients That Can Protect You from Respiratory Infection

Over the last couple of years, more and more research is coming to light about vitamin D. Not only is vitamin D considered to be one of the most important nutrients for healthy bones, but also it appears to keep the immune system healthy, which can protect the body from infection. Research suggests that vitamin D may help your body build and mount a proper defense against viruses and bacteria that can lead to pneumonia. You may be taking vitamin D already. If you are not taking vitamin D, you will want to supplement with 2,000 to 4,000 IU of vitamin D as a preventative. If you are in the hospital, I would recommend taking 4,000 to 10,000 IU per day; just make sure you are taking the natural vitamin D$_3$.

The second nutrient is called N-acetyl-cysteine (NAC). NAC helps to stimulate immune function, act as an antioxidant to the lungs, and thin out the mucus within the lungs to allow the defenses to clear out offending organisms. Research with NAC has shown it to be an effective tool in protecting seniors from the flu virus (and possibly other organisms). This nutrient is readily available and can be taken 1,000 mg twice daily. As always, be sure to inform your healthcare team of any supplements you are taking.

Water Intake

It is very common for people to become dehydrated in a hospital setting. It is important that you be especially diligent in preventing yourself from becoming dehydrated, as this can cause numerous problems that may predispose you to infection, clotting, and/or heart failure. As you become dehydrated, the mucous membranes within the lungs begin to dry out. When this happens, the lungs become susceptible to infection and inflammation.

If dehydration continues, the blood can thicken and become more difficult to circulate, which can promote heart failure. In addition, lack of fluid intake can lead to electrolyte imbalances that can cause the heart rhythm to change, again setting the stage for heart failure. Finally, thick blood has a tendency to clot easily. Blood clots are a major risk after surgery of the leg and hip; regular water consumption can be the first and most important step in preventing this blood clots from forming.

Final Thoughts:

If you are reading this report, I would imagine that you are either recently out of hip fracture surgery, have a family member who has suffered a hip fracture, or perceive yourself to be at high risk of hip fracture. My intention in writing this report is to provide you with the tools that you need to prevent such a situation and/or help you to improve your chances of surviving a hip fracture.

While researching the information for this report, I was surprised to see how sparse the research was for interventions designed to improve people's chances of surviving hip fractures. It appears that nobody seems to be interested in studying this major problem. I honestly believe that the recommendations within this report could have a significant effect on your recovery if you find yourself in the unfortunate situation of suffering a hip fracture; I implore you to take an active role in your own care.

Here are my recommendations:

1. Be proactive; get involved in the decision-making process.
2. Be squeaky; the squeaky wheel gets the grease. Politely demand excellence in your own care.
3. Be aggressive with your efforts to get better; decide to survive and thrive.
4. Be preemptive; do everything in your power to build strong bones; equally important, make your life "fall-proof."

20

Appendix A: The 18-Point Fracture Risk Checklist

The 18-Point Bone Quality Checklist:

1. Do you have poor distance depth perception? (If in doubt, check "yes.")
2. Do you have impaired vision? (Poor vision is a risk factor.)
3. Do you rarely exercise, such as walking or weight lifting? (Sedentary lifestyle is a major risk factor.)
4. Do you have low bone density? (This is *a* risk factor, not *the* risk factor.)

5. Do you take PPIs for reflux or heartburn? (This factor was not in the University of California study but has recently been shown to dramatically increase the risk of fracture.)
6. Do you have trouble getting out of a chair without using your arms? (If you cannot rise from a chair without swinging greatly or using your arms, put a check.)
7. Do you currently use anticonvulsant medications? (These can include Dilantin®, Neurontin®, Lyrica®, phenytoin, diazepam, etc.)
8. Has your mother had a hip fracture before age 80? (If she has had a fracture, but it occurred after age 80, then leave this blank.)
9. Have you ever been diagnosed with hyperthyroidism? (Hyperthyroidism involves having too much thyroid hormone. Do not confuse this with hypothyroidism, which involves too little thyroid hormone and is not considered a risk factor.)

10. Do you currently use any tranquilizers or mood-altering medications? (This classification includes long-acting benzodiazepines such as alprazolam, chlordiazepoxide, phenobarbital, and any medication that ends in "epam.")
11. Do you have a resting pulse of 80 beats per minute or higher? (Test by checking the pulse in your wrist for 20 seconds and multiplying by 3.)
12. Have you had any fractures since age 50? (This includes any fractures of a finger, toe, back, hip, etc.)
13. Would you consider yourself in poor health? (Be honest with this question; self-reported poor health is a significant risk factor.)
14. Are you on your feet less than 4 hours per day? (Be honest with this one, too. If you are seated or lying on a couch more than 20 hours a day, then put a check in the box.)
15. Are you a senior citizen? (Sorry, but age does matter, and it does count against you when determining your fracture risk. If you get a discount at

restaurants and movie theaters, then answer "yes" to this question.)
16. Do you weigh less today than you did at age 25? (If you weight the same or more than you did at 25, then do not check.)
17. Are you shorter than you were at age 25? (Shrinking is a sign of poor bone quality.)
18. Do you drink caffeinated beverages or use diet pills containing caffeine? (Caffeine causes calcium loss.)

Scoring Your Test

Once you have completed the checklist, add up all the check marks and fill in the number below:

Number of Checks: _____

Good Density/Good Quality

If you scored two checks or fewer *not including low bone density,* then your risk of having an osteoporotic fracture is 1.1 per 1,000 woman-years. This means that your risk of fracture is extremely low due to good density and good quality, Congratulations!

Good Density/Bad Quality

If you scored five checks or more *not including low bone density,* then your risk of having an osteoporotic fracture is 19 per 1,000 woman-years. This means you have normal bone density but poor bone quality. Fracture rates are 19 times higher for women with many of the listed risk factors even though their density may be normal.

Bad Density/Bad Quality

If you scored five checks or more and had low bone density in the osteoporosis range, then your risk of having an osteoporotic fracture is 32 per 1,000 woman-years of life. This group accounts for a full 32 percent of all hip fracture incidences, even though they only account for approximately 6 percent of the female population investigated in this study.

21

Apendix B: Best and Worst Foods For pH Balance

A + Foods

- Lentils
- Seaweed
- Sea vegetables
- Umeboshi Plums
- Onions
- Citrus Fruits
- Watermelon
- Raspberries
- Cashews
- Cantaloupe
- Ginger
- Endive

- Soy Sauce
- Asparagus
- Broccoli
- Honeydew
- Olive
- Mango

B + Foods

- Apple Cider Vinegar
- Almond Milk
- Primrose Oil
- Green Tea
- Herbs
- Sprouts
- Cherries
- Apples
- Peaches
- Cod Liver Oil
- Almonds
- Potato
- Peppers
- Cauliflower
- Pears
- Pumpkin
- Cabbage
- Collard Greens

- Avocados
- Blackberries
- Papaya

B Foods

- Oats
- Quinoa
- Wild Rice
- Brussels sprouts
- Beets
- Celery
- Squash
- Turnip greens
- Lettuce
- Apricots
- Chives
- Bananas
- Pineapple juice
- Raisins
- Grapes
- Strawberries
- Blueberries
- Spirulina
- Cucumbers
- Carrots
- Zucchini

C Foods

- Chicken eggs
- Millet
- Brown rice
- Curry
- Honey
- Yogurt
- Rice milk
- Goat cheese
- Spinach
- Fava beans
- Kidney beans
- Chutney
- Rhubarb
- Coconut
- Dates
- Figs
- Butter
- Cream
- Maple Syrup
- Dried fruit

D Foods

- Milk
- Aged cheeses

- Lamb
- Shell Fish
- White rice
- Split pea
- White beans
- Lima Beans
- Black tea
- Soy cheese

F Foods

- Pork
- Chicken
- Mussels
- Coffee
- Aspartame
- Casein
- Non-aged cheeses
- Corn
- Rye
- Oat bran
- Pecans
- Green pea
- Peanuts
- Cranberry
- Pomegranate

F- Foods

- Table salt
- Beer
- Soda
- Processed cheeses
- Ice cream
- Beef
- Lobster
- Brazil Nuts
- Fried Foods
- Spaghetti
- Soybean
- Sugar
- Yeast
- All refined pastas and grains

CPSIA information can be obtained
at www.ICGtesting.com
Printed in the USA
BVHW051909140423
662362BV00003B/155

9 781806 311583